BREEDING HORSES

Dr Mina C.G. Davies Morel BSc, PhD

Head of the Equine Group
Institute of Rural Sciences
University of Wales
Aberystwyth

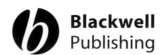

Blackwell
Publishing

© 2005 by Blackwell Publishing Ltd

Editorial Offices:
Blackwell Publishing Ltd, 9600 Garsington Road, Oxford OX4 2DQ, UK
   Tel: +44 (0)1865 776868
Blackwell Publishing Professional, 2121 State Avenue, Ames, Iowa 50014-8300,
USA
   Tel: +1 515 292 0140
Blackwell Publishing Asia, 550 Swanston Street, Carlton, Victoria 3053, Australia
   Tel: +61 (0)3 8359 1011

First published 2005 by Blackwell Publishing Ltd

Library of Congress Cataloging-in-Publication Data
Davies Morel, Mina C.G.
    Breeding horses / Mina C.G. Davies Morel.
       p.   cm.
    Includes bibliographical references and index.
    ISBN-10: 1-4051-2966-2 (pbk. : alk. paper)
    ISBN-13: 978-1-4051-2966-4 (pbk : alk. paper)
  1. Horses—Reproduction. 2. Horses—Breeding. I. Title.

    SF768.2.H67D38 2005
    636.1'082—dc22

                                            2005001818

ISBN-13 978-14051-2966-4
ISBN-10 1-4051-2966-2

A catalogue record for this title is available from the British Library

Set in 10 on 12.5 pt Palatino
by SNP Best-set Typesetter Ltd., Hong Kong
Printed and bound in India
by Replika Press Pvt, Ltd, Kundli

The publisher's policy is to use permanent paper from mills that operate a
sustainable forestry policy, and which has been manufactured from pulp
processed using acid-free and elementary chlorine-free practices. Furthermore,
the publisher ensures that the text paper and cover board used have met
acceptable environmental accreditation standards.

For further information on Blackwell Publishing, visit our website:
www.blackwellpublishing.com

Contents

Acknowledgements

I am most grateful to many people for their help and support in the preparation of this book. In particular I would like to thank all those that have kindly provided me with photographs or allowed me to take my own, and Alison Bramwell, Riceal Tully, Madeline Young and Shirley George for their diagrams. I would also like to thank CABI Publishing for their permission to reproduce the diagrams and photographs originally published by them (see individual figures for details). Lastly, but by no means least, I would like to thank my family for their continued support.

Dedication

This book is dedicated to my sons, Christopher and Andrew

Reproductive Anatomy

1.1 INTRODUCTION

A knowledge of reproductive anatomy and the control of reproduction will allow you to understand the reasons for many management and veterinary practices.

1.2 REPRODUCTIVE ANATOMY OF THE MARE

The mare's reproductive tract is a Y-shaped tubular organ. The perineum, vulva, vagina, and cervix form a series of seals protecting the more delicate, inner structures (the uterus, fallopian tubes and ovaries) which are responsible for producing gametes (the unfertilised eggs or *ova*), fertilisation and embryo development (Figures 1.1, 1.2 and 1.3).

1.2.1 The vulva and perineum

The vulva (Figures 1.1 and 1.3) is the outer part of the reproductive system, protecting the entrance to the vagina. Either side of the vulva lie the vulval lips which should touch, forming a seal. Below the entrance to the vagina, in the lower part of the vulva, lie the clitoris and the surrounding clitoral sinuses. These are important in the mare as they provide an ideal environment for the collection and growth of bacteria such as those which cause venereal disease and subsequent infertility. This area is therefore swabbed to test for bacteria before covering. In the thoroughbred industry such swabbing is compulsory (Section 3.4.1). The clitoral area is also important as one of the signs of oestrous in a mare (i.e. ready for mating) is the opening and closing of the vulval lips to expose the clitoris, a process referred to as 'winking' (Figure 2.3, p. 42).

The perineum is the name given to the area around the vulva and anus. Good conformation of this area is important as the area protects the reproductive tract from bacterial invasion. Poor conformation

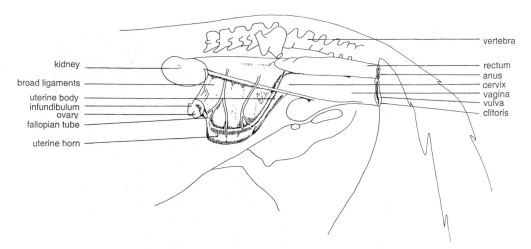

kidney

broad ligaments

uterine body
infundibulum
ovary
fallopian tube

uterine horn

vertebra

rectum
anus
cervix
vagina
vulva
clitoris

Figure 1.1   A lateral (side) view of the reproductive tract of the mare. © CABI.

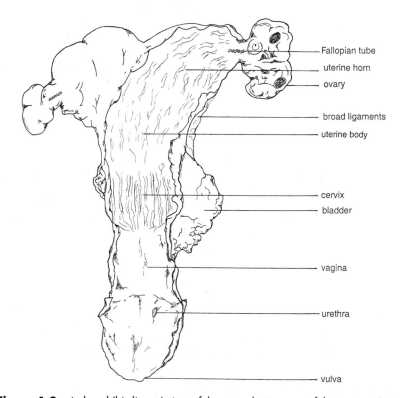

Fallopian tube
uterine horn
ovary

broad ligaments
uterine body

cervix
bladder

vagina

urethra

vulva

Figure 1.2   A dorsal (bird's eye) view of the reproductive tract of the mare. © CABI.

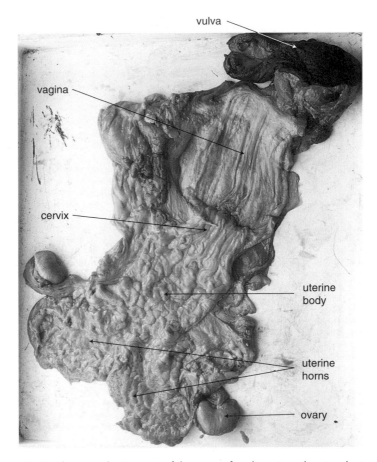

vulva

vagina

cervix

uterine body

uterine horns

ovary

Figure 1.3 The reproductive tract of the mare after dissection, showing the internal surfaces of the tract. The vulva is at the top right, below which is the vagina collapsed followed by the cervix lined by distinct folds, followed by the uterus with its less distinct endometrial folds and lastly the ovaries at bottom left and right. © CABI.

leads to air being sucked in and out of the vagina (*pneumovagina*) as the mare moves. There is a risk that along with the air, bacteria and faeces may also pass into the vagina (Figure 1.4). If this occurs the levels of bacteria will eventually be so high that they will pass through the cervix and on into the uterus causing a uterine infection (*endometritis*) which can lead to permanent infertility.

1.2.2 Protection of the genital tract

Adequate protection of the reproductive tract is essential to prevent uterine infection (endometritis). The tract has three seals: the vulval seal, the vaginal seal and the cervix (Figure 1.5).

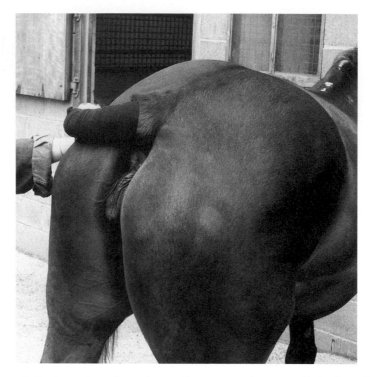

Figure 1.4   A poorly conformed mare showing a sunken anus which allows faeces to collect on the vulva and, along with air, pass into the reproductive tract and so cause uterine infections. © CABI.

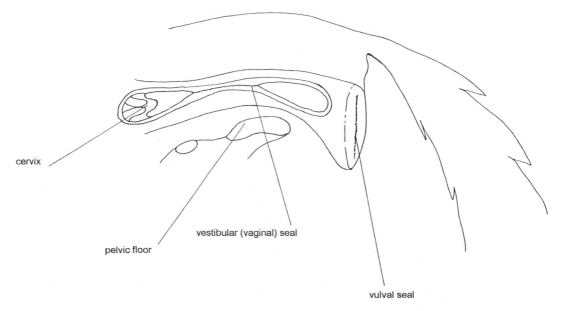

Figure 1.5   The three 'seals' in the reproductive tract of the mare. © CABI.

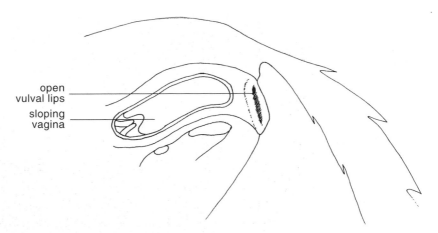

Figure 1.6 A poorly conformed mare showing vulval lips which fail to form a seal, a sunken anus and a vagina which slopes downwards internally. Such a mare is at severe risk of uterine infection from both airborne bacteria passing into the tract and from contamination from faeces falling onto the vulva from the sunken anus above.

The vulval seal is outermost and is formed by the closeness of the vulval lips. The vaginal seal is formed by the walls of the vagina naturally sticking together as they rest on the pelvis. The final seal is formed by the tight muscle of the cervix. In a mare with good conformation these seals provide protection from bacteria. However, poor conformation prevents these seals from working correctly. In the worst cases of poor conformation the vulval lips fail to meet and the anus is sunken in, which allows faeces to collect on the vulva. In addition the vagina may slope downwards towards the cervix thereby preventing infections from draining out naturally (Figures 1.4 and 1.6).

Poor perineal and vulval conformation is most commonly seen in mares in athletic, lean condition, such as thoroughbred mares, and also in older mares which have had several foals (*multiparous*). It can be helped by a Caslick's vulvoplasty operation, in which the lips of the top 50–70% of the vulva are cut, and the two sides then sewn together. The two raw edges heal, as in the healing of an open wound, and seal the upper part of the vulva, preventing faeces passing into the vagina (Figure 1.7 a–c). A hole is left at the bottom of the vulva for urine but is often not big enough to allow the mare to be mated except by artificial insemination (AI). For natural mating the area usually has to be cut open before and re-sewn after mating, and always cut for foaling.

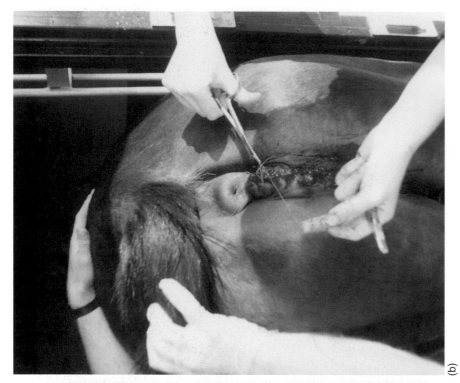

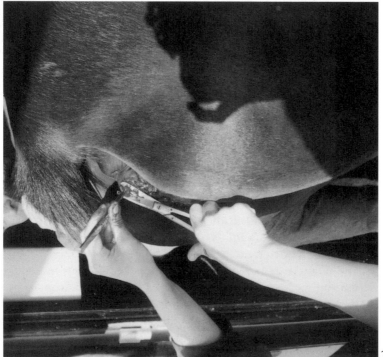

Figure 1.7 (a)–(c) A Caslick's operation in the mare showing; (a) the cutting of the vulval lips; (b) suturing; and (c) the finished job. © CABI.

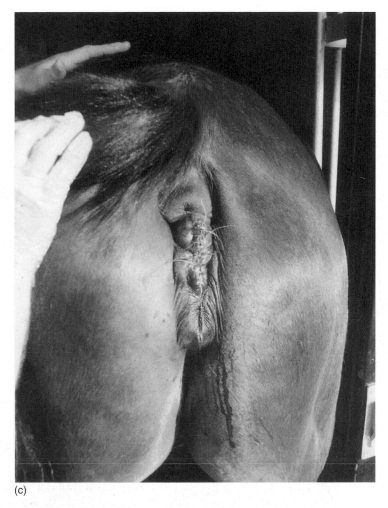

(c)

Figure 1.7 (a)–(c)   *(cont'd)*

1.2.3 The vagina

The vagina lies between the vulva and the cervix. It forms part of the outer protective reproductive tract and is supported by the pelvis. The walls are normally collapsed and form the vaginal seal, though it can expand remarkably to allow the foal to pass through at birth (*parturition*). The secretions in the vagina are acidic and as bacteria cannot survive in acid conditions, these secretions also help to prevent infection. However, sperm are also unable to survive in acidic conditions and so at mating sperm are deposited into the top of the cervix/bottom of the uterus to avoid the vagina. The urethra passes from the bladder and opens into the *caudal* (tail end) vagina.

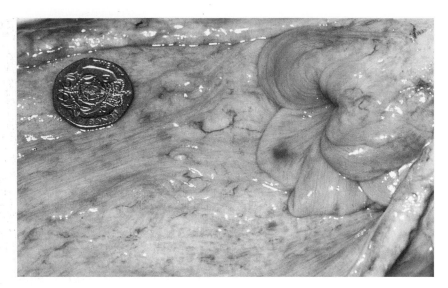

Figure 1.8   The cervix and internal surface of the vagina in the mare, showing the cervix relaxed and 'flowering' into the vagina. © CABI.

1.2.4 The cervix

The cervix is a tight, thick-walled muscle at the entrance to the uterus. When the mare is sexually inactive, during dioestrus (Section 2.2.1.1.1, p. 38) or pregnant, the cervix is tightly closed and appears white with thick secretions making it a very effective seal. When the mare is sexually active, during oestrus, the cervix relaxes and appears to 'flower' into the vagina, its colour is pink with thinner secretions (Figure 1.8). This makes it easier for the sperm to be deposited into the cervix/uterus. The cervix is lined by a series of folds which are continuous with folds in the uterus (Figure 1.3, p. 3) and allows the cervix to expand (*dilate*) greatly at parturition.

1.2.5 The uterus

The uterus is a hollow muscular organ supported by the broad ligaments which attach it to the vertebra and provide support. The uterus is divided into two, the body and the horns (Figures 1.1 and 1.2, p. 2). The exact size of the uterus varies but generally the body is a little bigger than the horns. The body of the uterus is bigger than in many other livestock as the mare carries one fetus which lies mainly within the uterine body. The walls of the uterus, like those of the vagina, are

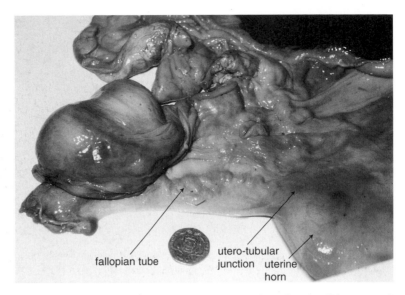

Figure 1.9 The convoluted fallopian tube running from the top of the uterine horn (bottom right) to the ovary (left). The utero-tubular junction area can be seen where the large uterine horn abruptly reduces down in size to the small convoluted fallopian tube. © CABI.

collapsed down upon each other in the non-pregnant mare and lie intermingled with the intestines. The uterine wall consists of three layers: a) outer connective tissue layer, which provides support; b) a middle muscle layer, which allows expansion as the foal grows and contraction at parturition; and c) inner endometrium, arranged in folds and the site of attachment for the placenta. *Endometritis* (infection or inflammation of the endometrium) can be a serious condition, often leading to infertility.

1.2.6 The fallopian tubes

The mare has two fallopian tubes (*oviducts*) connecting the top of each uterine horn with each ovary. The junction between the fallopian tube and the uterus is called the *utero-tubular junction* (Figure 1.9).

Each fallopian tube is about 5mm in diameter and highly convoluted (Figure 1.9). Fertilisation occurs towards the ovary end of the fallopian tube in an area called the *ampulla*. In the mare all ova are released from one specific area of the ovary called the ovulation fossa, they are then caught by the *infundibulum* and funnelled into the fallopian tube to await fertilisation. The infundibulum is a 'scrunched-

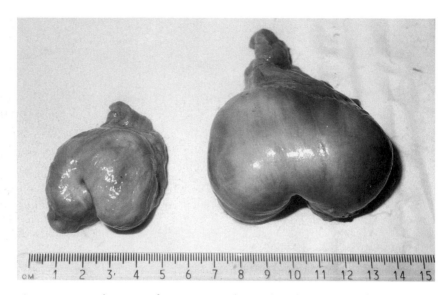

Figure 1.10   The ovaries from a mare in the non breeding season (left) and breeding season (right). Note the bean-shape and the ovulation fossa in the centre of the concave surface. © CABI.

up' funnel shape at the end of the fallopian tube and is attached to one area of the ovary, the *ovulation fossa*.

1.2.7 The ovaries

The ovaries of the mare are responsible for producing gametes (ova) for fertilisation and the hormones which control reproductive activity. They are bean-shaped and about 4–8 cm × 4–6 cm in size during the breeding season (Figures 1.10 and 1.11).

The whole ovary, except for the ovulation fossa, is contained within a protective layer or fibrous capsule, and all development of the ova occurs inside the ovary within this protective covering (Figure 1.12).

1.2.7.1 Follicular development and ovulation

The number of potential ova contained within the ovary is determined before birth, and at this stage the ova are immature and termed *oogonia*, and there are many more than an individual mare will use in her reproductive lifetime. Each oogonia as it develops is contained within a follicle. The follicle is initially just a simple layer of cells surrounding the oogonia, but as the oogonia develops into an ova and on to ovulation, these cells secrete fluid and the follicle becomes a

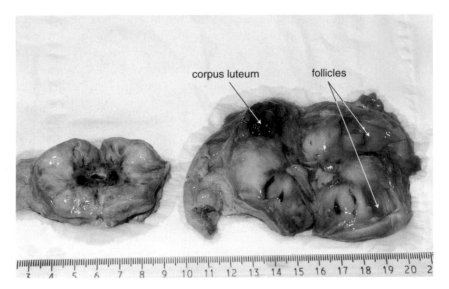

Figure 1.11 A cross-section taken through the two ovaries shown in Figure 1.10. Note in the active ovary (on the right) a corpus luteum (dark red mass at the top left) and a large follicle (hollow or space at the top right) and smaller follicle (bottom right). © CABI.

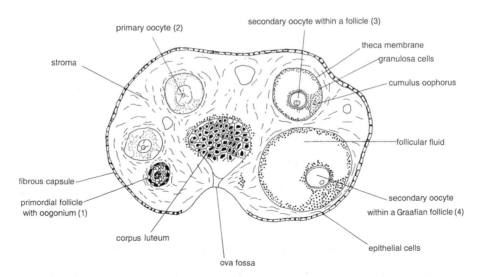

Figure 1.12 Diagrammatic representation of follicular development (1)–(4) and ovulation within the ovary (not to scale). © CABI.

fluid-filled structure within the ovary. The initial simple follicle containing the oogonia, with its full number of chromosomes (64), is termed a *primordial follicle*. At birth, the ovary contains many thousands of these. After birth, and before puberty, some of these oogonia start to develop into *primary oocytes*, the name given to the oogonia undergoing the first stages of meiosis. Meiosis is a particular type of cell division which occurs in the ovaries or testes specifically to produce the ovum and the sperm. During meiosis the parent cells, which have a full (*diploid*) number of chromosomes (64 chromosomes in the horse), divide into the ovum or sperm which have half the full number of chromosomes (*haploid*, 32 chromosomes in the horse). At fertilisation the haploid number of chromosomes in the ovum fuses with the haploid in the sperm to give a fertilised ovum with the full number of chromosomes (diploid). The primary oocytes then remain dormant until puberty, when hormone secretion associated with the oestrous cycle drives them to develop further.

From puberty onwards these primary oocytes develop and complete the final stages of meiosis at varying rates providing a regular supply of ova ready for *ovulation* (when the ova are released for fertilisation) every 21 days during the breeding season. As each follicle develops its cells secrete follicular fluid, which fills the cavity surrounding the oocyte. As the follicle grows, more fluid accumulates; most follicles reach about 3 cm in diameter before ovulation, though some may be much bigger. Not all primary oocytes go on to develop fully, many are lost and normally only one reaches the stage ready for ovulation in any one 21-day cycle. The fully developed follicle is now called a *Graafian follicle* (Figure 1.12).

Ovulation, or release, of the Graafian follicle is triggered by a hormone called luteinising hormone or LH (Section 2.2.1.1.1, p. 38). This hormone causes the follicle to collapse and the ovum plus follicular fluid to be released through the ovulation fossa into the infundibulum and then passed down the fallopian tube for possible fertilisation. In the mare normally only one ovum is released per oestrous period though increasingly in some breeds more than one ovulation is seen (this is known as *multiple ovulation*) which may represent a big problem to the mare (Section 5.4, p. 119).

After the release of the ovum and follicular fluid, the old follicle collapses and bleeding occurs into the centre of the cavity left behind, forming a blood clot. This clot is called the *corpus luteum* (CL or yellow body) (Figures 1.11 and 1.12). Initially the CL is reddish-purple in colour, as it ages and becomes inactive it becomes smaller and brown, then finally white in colour. The role of the CL is to secrete progesterone, the hormone of pregnancy. For as long as the CL is active, progesterone will be secreted and the mare will not return to oestrus (Section 2.2.1.1.1, p. 38).

1.3 REPRODUCTIVE ANATOMY OF THE STALLION

The stallion's reproductive tract can be divided into two areas, the outer part responsible for depositing semen (*sperm* and *seminal plasma*), and the inner part responsible for producing hormones, gametes (sperm) and supporting fluid (seminal plasma) (Figures 1.13 and 1.14).

1.3.1 The penis

The penis of the stallion may be divided into the glans penis, the body or shaft, and the roots. In the resting position the penis lies held within the sheath and out of sight.

The area within the sheath (*prepuce*) is the glans penis (*rose*). The sheath (Figure 1.13) provides protection to this sensitive area. At the end of the glans penis is the opening of the urethra. The folds of

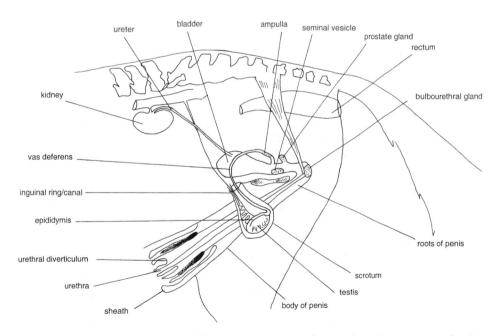

Figure 1.13 A lateral (side) view of the reproductive tract of the stallion (the penis area has been enlarged for clarity).

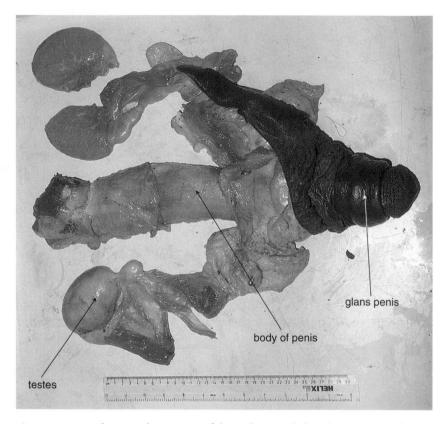

glans penis

body of penis

testes

Figure 1.14 The reproductive tract of the stallion (excluding the accessory glands) after dissection, illustrating the glans penis (right), the main body of the penis (centre) and the testes (bottom left, dissected top left). © CABI.

the sheath retain dirt and old cellular material (*smegma*) and provide an ideal, warm, moist environment for the collection and growth of bacteria. As is seen in the mare, these bacteria may be responsible for venereal disease (VD), which can cause infertility in the mare. This area is, therefore, regularly swabbed to test for bacteria prior to covering; again in the thoroughbred industry such swabbing is compulsory (Section 3.5.1, p. 76). The glans penis, like the body of the penis, contains erectile tissue which is haemodynamic (i.e. reacts to increasing blood pressure). The glans penis also contains extra erectile tissue which allows it to increase further in size at erection.

The majority of erectile tissue is within the body of the penis (Figure 1.15) and mainly in an area called the *corpus carvernosum penis*, which is the largest area of the penis, and is contained within a fibrous capsule, the *tunica albuginea*. This capsule provides support, but also limits the increase in size at erection. A much smaller area of erectile

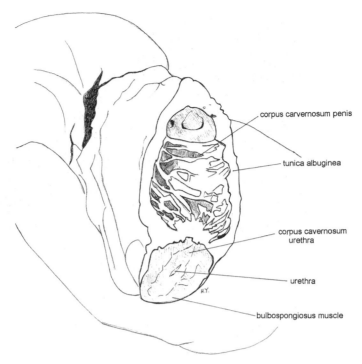

corpus carvernosum penis

tunica albuginea

corpus cavernosum urethra

urethra

bulbospongiosus muscle

Figure 1.15 Cross-section through the main body of the penis of the stallion. © CABI.

tissue (*corpus carvernosum urethra*) is found around the urethra which is also surrounded by the bulbospongiosus muscle.

The roots attach the penis to the pelvis via ligaments and it is in this area that the *vas deferens* ducts join with the urethra from the bladder. The urethra then runs between the two roots, into the body of the penis and exits at the glans penis (Figure 1.13).

The process of depositing semen into the mare's reproductive tract involves erection and ejaculation. Erection is the term given to the increase in penis size, which occurs in response to a mare in oestrous or other form of sexual stimulation such as the sight of an AI dummy, or covering yard. This causes arousal and an increase in blood flow to the erectile tissue of the penis. The increase in blood pressure results in an increase in size (*erection*). Ejaculation then follows, causing the sperm to pass from the testes along the vas deferens, past the accessory glands where seminal plasma is added, and exited via the urethra. This movement of sperm is caused by contraction of the muscle walls of the vas deferens, urethra and the penis. Semen normally exits in six to nine jets, the initial three contain the majority of the sperm.

1.3.2 The accessory glands

The accessory glands are a series of four glands situated between the end of the vas deferens and the roots of the penis (Figure 1.13). The glands nearest the penis are the bulbourethral glands, followed by the prostate gland, the seminal vesicles and lastly the ampulla glands at the end of the vas deferens. Together these glands secrete seminal plasma, the fluid part of semen, which helps transport the sperm along the stallion's tract and into the mare. Seminal plasma also causes the final development of the sperm in preparation for fertilisation and provides the energy and nutrients required for sperm survival.

1.3.3 The vas deferens

The stallion has two vas deferens which connect each testis to the single urethra (Figure 1.13). Their role is to transport sperm from the testes, to join with the urethra. Each vas deferens has a thick muscular wall which contracts, propelling sperm along. The lumen (diameter) of the duct is small and near to the testes it is highly folded, which increases its surface area and so increases the area available for sperm storage.

1.3.4 The testes

The testes of the stallion, as with the ovaries of the mare, are responsible for producing gametes (sperm) for fertilisation, and hormones to control reproductive activity. They hang outside the body cavity and each is connected to the main body via the inguinal canal (Figures 1.16 and 1.17). The inguinal canal contains the vas deferens along with the nerve supply, blood vessels and an area of muscle called the cremaster muscle.

The testes lie outside the stallion's body and this allows a temperature of 35–36°C (3°C below body temperature) to be maintained. Sperm production (*spermatogenesis*) is maximised at this lower temperature, so any increases in environmental temperature result in a decrease in spermatogenesis. The temperature of the testes is controlled by the cremaster muscle, the large number of scrotal sweat glands and the pampiniform plexus. The cremaster muscle contracts in response to cold, fear etc. and so draws the testes up closer to the body thereby helping to maintain the temperature, in hot weather it relaxes allowing the testes to be carried lower and so cooled more effectively. The sweat glands also help cooling in hot weather. The pampiniform plexus is a counter-current, heat exchange system between the artery entering the testes and the vein leaving it (Figure

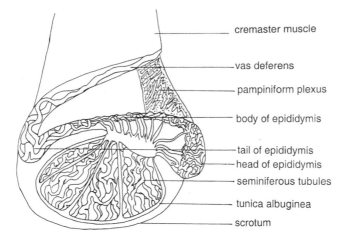

cremaster muscle

vas deferens

pampiniform plexus

body of epididymis

tail of epididymis
head of epididymis
seminiferous tubules

tunica albuginea

scrotum

Figure 1.16 A lateral (side) view of the testis of the stallion. © CABI.

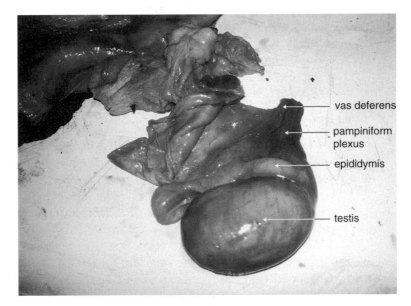

vas deferens

pampiniform plexus

epididymis

testis

Figure 1.17 A dissected stallion testis, illustrating the main body of the testis, the epididymis, pampiniform plexus and vas deferens. © CABI.

1.16). Both the artery entering and the vein leaving the testes divide into a fine capillary network, in which they come into close contact (*pampiniform plexus*). This closeness allows an exchange of heat from the warm artery entering the testes to the cooler vein leaving. As the heat moves from the artery to the vein, the artery cools down in readiness to enter the testes and the vein heats up ready to enter the body.

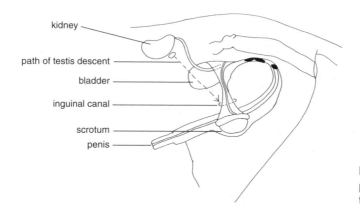

kidney

path of testis descent

bladder

inguinal canal

scrotum

penis

Figure 1.18 The normal passage of descent of testes in the stallion. © CABI.

The testes lie within a skin covering, the scrotum, into which they drop either just before birth or soon afterwards (Figure 1.18). Occasionally one or both testes fail to descend fully in which case the stallion is called a *cryptorchid* or *rig*. Such animals can be mistaken for geldings, but, if the testes are lying just above the inguinal canal they may still be capable of producing some sperm plus hormones. The animal is, therefore, likely to show stallion behaviour and may be capable of fertilising a mare.

Lying over the top of the testes is the *epididymis* (Figure 1.16), a series of long convoluted tubules. The epididymis connects the testes to the vas deferens but also stores sperm ready for ejaculation, reabsorbs fluid and drives further sperm maturation. This maturation is essential so that sperm, after mixing with seminal plasma, are ready for the final stage maturation (*capacitation*) in the female tract. The epididymis also reabsorbs any sperm not ejaculated, ensuring a continual supply of fresh sperm.

The main part of the testis is divided into seminiferous tubules and surrounding intertubular spaces (Figure 1.19). Each area has a specific function, the seminiferous tubules and the Sertoli cells within them are responsible for sperm production, the intertubular spaces, containing the Leydig cells, are responsible for hormone (particularly testosterone) production.

1.3.4.1 Sperm and spermatogenesis

The Sertoli cells lining the seminiferous tubules act as nurse cells, nourishing and supporting the developing spermatozoa. In a similar manner to the mare's ova, sperm start as undeveloped germ cells or spermatogonia attached to the wall of the seminiferous tubules. They then undergo spermatogenesis as they progressively develop, by

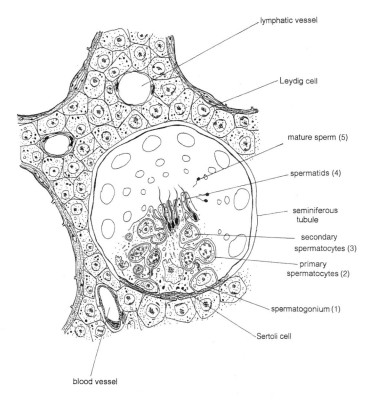

Figure 1.19 A cross-section through an area of the testis of the stallion, illustrating a seminiferous tubule with the gradual development of spermatogonia to mature spermatids, and the intertubular spaces. © CABI.

meiosis, into mature sperm. They develop attached to the same Sertoli cell throughout their development, i.e. do not switch from Sertoli cell to Sertoli cell as they develop but stick to the same one, (Figure 1.19) and are eventually released into the lumen of the seminiferous tubule and make their way to the epididymis. Spermatogenesis in the stallion takes 57 days and occurs continuously, ensuring a ready supply of mature sperm. Unlike the mare, the stallion does not have a finite number of sperm per lifetime, new cells continually develop into spermatogonia ready to undergo spermatogenesis. The average daily production of a mature stallion is $7–8 \times 10^9$ (7000–8000 million) sperm.

Sperm structurally consist of three areas: the head, the mid-piece and the tail (Figure 1.20), with three distinct functions.

The sperm head contains the DNA in the chromosomes, these are haploid in number (32, i.e. half the normal number of 64) to allow them to fuse with the ovum (also haploid) to give the normal diploid complement (64 being the full number). At the top of the sperm head is

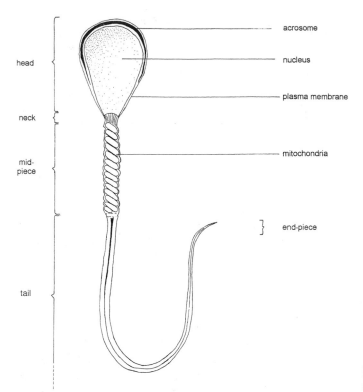

head

neck

mid-piece

tail

acrosome

nucleus

plasma membrane

mitochondria

end-piece

Figure 1.20 A typical stallion sperm. © CABI.

the acrosome region. This area fuses with the ova membrane and is important in fertilisation.

The mid-piece of the sperm contains mainly mitochondria, organelles within the cell which produce energy. The mid-piece is often termed the 'power plant' of the sperm, as it provides the energy to drive the tail.

The tail is made up of a series of muscle fibres which are driven by the energy provided by the mid-piece, causing the tail to whip from side to side propelling the sperm forwards and producing a wave-like motion.

1.3.4.2 Semen

Semen is the term given to seminal plasma plus sperm, and in the stallion is a milky-white, thick fluid. The volume varies between stallions and with stallion age and time of year, but is normally 30–250 ml (Table 1.1), though a significant amount of this (up to 80 ml) may be gel, which forms a thick jelly-like layer on the top of a semen sample if it is left to stand for a while. This gel layer contains no sperm, it is the remaining sperm-rich fraction which is important for fertilisation.

Table 1.1 Average seminal characteristics in the stallion.

Component	Normal value
Volume	30–250 ml
Gel fraction	0–80 ml
Sperm concentration	$30–600 \times 10^6\,\mathrm{ml}^{-1}$
Total number of sperm/ejaculation	$900 \times 10^6–150 \times 10^9$

1.4 PREGNANCY

The anatomy of pregnancy in the mare can be divided into three main sections: fertilisation, embryo development and placenta development.

1.4.1 Fertilisation

The ovum waits for the sperm in the ampulla of the fallopian tube. The sperm move towards the fallopian tubes as a result of contractions in the mare's tract and the driving action of their own tails. They are also attracted by chemicals produced by the ova. As the sperm pass up through the mare's tract the uterine secretions cause capacitation, which activates enzymes in the acrosome region of the sperm head ready for fertilisation.

By means of the whipping action of their tails and the enzymes released at capacitation the sperm force their way through the outer gelatinous layer of the ovum and then the zona pellucida (jelly layer surrounding the ovum) (Figure 1.21).

As the sperm head meets the membrane of the ovum the two fuse. The nuclei of the sperm and the ovum then unite, joining their two haploid complements (32) of chromosomes to give the full diploid (64) of the new individual. This newly combined genetic material now dictates all the characteristics of the new individual.

After fertilisation the ovum is now termed a *conceptus* and at five to six days after fertilisation passes out of the fallopian tube through the utero-tubular junction to the uterus, where it remains for the rest of pregnancy.

1.4.2 Embryo development

Twenty-four hours after mating, the conceptus, now termed a *zygote*, has divided by *mitosis* (growth by cell division) into two cells. It continues to divide into 4, 16, 32 cells etc. and at four days old it is a bundle of cells known as the *morula* (Figure 1.21).

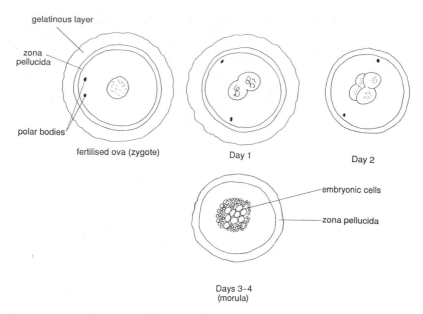

gelatinous layer

zona pellucida

polar bodies

fertilised ova (zygote)

Day 1

Day 2

embryonic cells

zona pellucida

Days 3–4
(morula)

Figure 1.21 The stages of development from fertilised ovum (zygote) to morula in the equine conceptus. © CABI.

The cells continue to divide and the morula moves to the uterotubular junction. At Day 5–6 it passes through this junction into the uterus. At this stage it is important that the uterus is in a fit condition to accept the embryo. At Day 5 a thin capsule appears around the morula (Figures 1.22 and 1.23) which protects it, keeping it in its clear spherical shape and allowing it to move freely within the uterus during early pregnancy. All equine concepti go through this period of mobility (free living) which is essential to let the uterus know that there is a pregnancy within. From Day 6 the morula continues to grow (Figure 1.23) and now relies on uterine secretions for all its nutrients as it floats freely within the uterus.

At Day 8 the cells of the morula become organised into three groups: the *embryonic disc* (the embryo), the *blastocoel* (a temporary nutrient store) and the *trophoblast* (future placenta) (Figure 1.23). The morula is now termed a *blastocyst*. This cell organisation marks the beginning of the switching on and off of various genes within cells; these cells then become destined to develop along set paths. Before this each cell was in theory capable of developing into a new individual as none of its genes had been switched off.

Further organisation then takes place and three different cell layers appear within the blastocyst, which form different parts of the embryo and placenta by Day 14. These layers are called the ectoderm, meso-

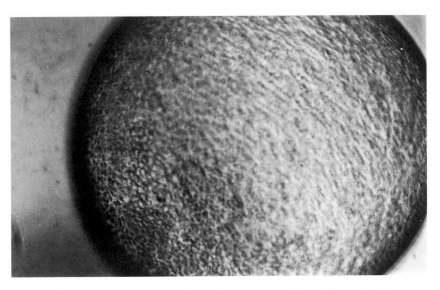

Figure 1.22 A view of the surface of an equine embryo, illustrating the outer trophoblast surface cells. The capsule can be seen as a clear area encircling the whole conceptus (bottom and top right). (Photograph courtesy of Alison Crook, © CABI.)

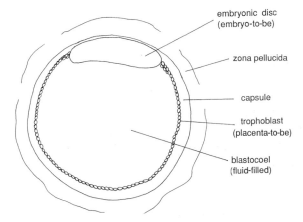

embryonic disc
(embryo-to-be)

zona pellucida

capsule

trophoblast
(placenta-to-be)

blastocoel
(fluid-filled)

Figure 1.23 The equine blastocyst at Day 8 after fertilisation, showing the capsule and the organisation of three areas: embryonic disc, blastocoel and trophoblast. © CABI.

derm and endoderm. In the placenta they form the attachment to the uterus (*ectoderm*), the blood supply (*mesoderm*) and the inner surface (*endoderm*). In the embryo they form the skin and outer layers (ectoderm), the blood vessels and muscle blocks (mesoderm), and the internal systems (circulatory, gastro-intestinal systems etc.) (endoderm).

At this stage the layers which will go to form the placenta now form the yolk sac wall. Nutrients from the uterus pass across this to be stored in the blastocoel or yolk sac to be used by the embryo as needed.

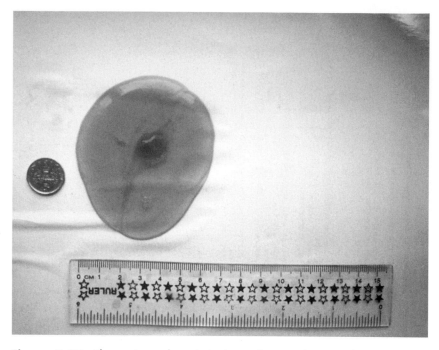

Figure 1.24 The equine embryo is a clear sphere in shape, making it easy to identify at an early stage using an ultrasonic scanner.

Throughout its early development the embryo is a clear sphere in shape, this means that, like the human embryo but unlike in the cow and ewe, it can be identified easily at an early stage using an ultrasonic scanner (Figure 1.24, and Section 5.35, p. 118).

At Day 16 the placental tissue starts to fold around the embryo to enclose a fluid-filled protective space; this forms the amnion containing the amniotic fluid (Figure 1.25). Initially, it can be seen as a clear, fluid-filled bubble (Figure 1.26) though in time it collapses around the fetus at a later stage. Throughout pregnancy the amnion provides a clean, protective environment in which the embryo can develop. The volume of amniotic fluid at foaling is 3.5 litres.

Until Day 18–20 the conceptus is free living (mobility phase) within the uterus, after this its movements slow down as it starts to attach to the uterine wall. As the attachment gets stronger the conceptus stops moving altogether.

As the embryo grows within the conceptus specific areas can gradually be identified. At Day 12 the head and tail end can be seen. At Day 15 the future muscle blocks and central nervous system (CNS) are evident. By Day 23 all the basic bodily structures are present though

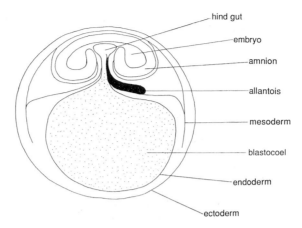

- hind gut
- embryo
- amnion
- allantois
- mesoderm
- blastocoel
- endoderm
- ectoderm

Figure 1.25 The development of the equine placenta at Day 20 after fertilisation, showing the development of the allantoic sac. © CABI.

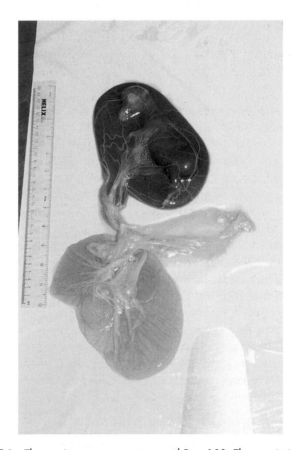

Figure 1.26 The equine conceptus at around Day 100. The amniotic sac forming a bubble of fluid around the embryo can be seen along with the placenta (bottom). The dark appearance of the amniotic fluid is due to changes post mortem, it would normally be clear.

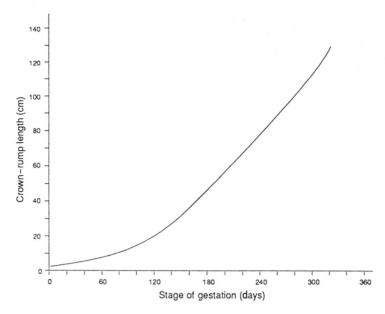

Figure 1.27 The increase in fetal crown–rump length during gestation. © CABI.

only in an undeveloped form. The embryo by this time has taken on its characteristic 'C' shape and lies away from the placenta attached only by the umbilical cord. The tail, CNS, head, brain areas, pharynx, gut and body muscle can all now be seen. From now on development is the fine growth and organisation of these undeveloped areas. By Day 40 all the main body features are evident e.g. limbs, tail, nostrils, pigmented eyes, ears, elbow and stifle regions, eyelids, etc. and the embryo is now termed a fetus. At Day 39–45 the sex of the fetus is determined and is evident from the external appearance. Once development is complete increase in growth occurs (Figure 1.27). The main milestones in equine fetal development are summarised in Table 1.2.

Full term sees the birth of a well developed foal with all the characteristics typical of an animal which has evolved to survive on open plains and escapes from its predators by outrunning them. Within 30 to 60 minutes of birth foals are capable of all basic bodily functions including walking and are, therefore, able to escape predators.

1.4.3 Development of the placenta

The placenta provides protection for the fetus and, after the mobility phase, a means both of getting nutrients and oxygen from the mare and of passing waste products back. The placenta develops from the

Table 1.2 A summary of the major milestones for fetal development through gestation. Reproduced with permission from CABI.

Day of gestation	Major development milestones
1	Zygote, 2 cells
4	Morula, 16 plus cells
5	Capsule formation
6	Hatching of morula
8	Blastocyst, differentiated into embryo, blastocoel and trophoblast
9	Ectoderm and endoderm germ layers evident
11	Caudal (tail) and cranial (head) ends of embryo evident
14	Mesoderm evident
16	Folds leading to the formation of the amnion can be seen, first blood vessels evident in mesoderm, conceptus 1.6–2 cm diameter
18	Fetus begins to take on characteristic 'C' shape
20	Allantois forming from outpushings of the fetal hindgut, conceptus is 3–4 cm diameter, eye vesicle and ear present, capsule around conceptus begins to degenerate
21	Amnion complete
23	All basic bodily structures evident, though in rudimentary state
25	Chorionic girdle first evident, attachment of fetus
26	Forelimb bud seen, three branchial arches present, eye visible
30	Genital tubercle present, eye lens seen
36	Rudimentary three digits seen on hoof, facial clefts closing, eyes pigmented and acoustic groove forming
40	Endometrial cups forming, ear forming, nostrils seen, eyelids seen, all limbs evident and elbow and stifle joint areas identifiable, conceptus is 6–7 cm diameter
42	Ear triangle in shape, mammary buds seen along ridge
45	External genitalia evident, allantoic sac volume 110 ml
47	Palate fused
49	Mammary teats evident
55	Ear covers acoustic groove, eyelids closing
60	Conceptus is 10–13 cm in diameter
63	Eyelids fused, fine eye development occurring, hoof, sole and frog areas of hoof evident
75	Female clitoris prominent
80	Scrotum clearly seen
90	Endometrial cups degenerate
95	Hoof appears yellow in colour
112	Tactile hairs on lips growing
120	Fine hair on muzzle, chin and eyelashes beginning to grow, eye prominent and ergot evident
150	Full attachment of placental microcotyledons, eyelashes clearly seen, enlargement of mammary gland
180	Mane and tail evident
240	Hair of poll, ears, chin, muzzle and throat evident
270	Whole of body covered with fine hair, longer mane and tail hair clearly seen
310	Allantoic sac volume 8.5 litres
320	Testes may drop from this time onwards
320–340	Birth of fully developed fetus

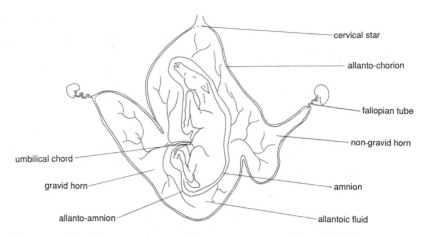

cervical star

allanto-chorion

fallopian tube

non-gravid horn

umbilical chord

gravid horn

amnion

allanto-amnion

allantoic fluid

Figure 1.28 The equine fetus and placenta near parturition. © CABI.

outer trophoblast of the conceptus. Initially the embryo obtains nutrients from the uterine secretions which pass to the blastocoel where they are stored ready for use. Soon this system cannot satisfy the demands of the embryo and so the conceptus loses its capsule and attaches to the uterine wall (Day 20–25) and begins to obtain nutrients directly from the mare. Waste products are passed back but also start to collect in the allantois, a sac which develops from the hind gut of the embryo (Figure 1.25).

The allantois increases in size with the embryo eventually surrounding it and dominating the conceptus. Eventually the embryo will be attached to the placenta by just the umbilical cord. The allantoic fluid is the straw-coloured 'waters' which are released at foaling, at which stage they are around 8.5 litres (Figure 1.28).

There are three attachment stages in the development of the placenta in the mare. The first, a loose temporary attachment, is the *chorionic girdle*, followed at Day 38 by the *endometrial cups*. These endometrial cups also secrete equine chorionic gonadotropin (eCG), sometimes referred to as pregnant mare serum gonadotropin (PMSG), a hormone essential in ensuring that the mare keeps her early pregnancy (Section 2.2.2.1, p. 48). From Day 90 the endometrial cups are gradually replaced by the placenta. Over time the placenta takes on a velvety appearance created by fine microvilli (hair-like projections) over its entire surface. These microvilli organise themselves into microscopic bundles (*microcotyledons*) which push into microscopic pockets in the uterine epithelium. This attachment takes until Day 150 to be fully complete (Figure 1.29).

The equine placenta is relatively thick with six cell layers (three on the fetal side and three on the maternal side). It is attached to the whole

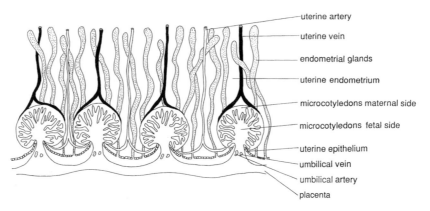

uterine artery
uterine vein
endometrial glands
uterine endometrium
microcotyledons maternal side
microcotyledons fetal side
uterine epithelium
umbilical vein
umbilical artery
placenta

Figure 1.29 The fully developed placenta of the mare. © CABI.

of the surface of the uterus and allows the mare's blood system to come close to the fetal blood system at the microcotyledons and so allows the transfer of nutrients and waste products. However, a thick placenta, such as in the mare, has the disadvantage of limiting the passage of large molecules. Some of the most important large molecules are proteins, in particular antibodies. There are two main ways in which young receive antibodies from their mother, either across the placenta during pregnancy or via colostrum immediately after birth (*parturition*). As the mare's placenta is so thick very few antibodies can pass from the mare to the fetus during pregnancy, so in the foal the antibodies passed via colostrum are vital to the foal's survival. The thickness of the placenta varies in other mammals, but in general, the thicker the placenta, the fewer antibodies pass across in pregnancy and the greater the importance of colostrum. At parturition the placenta of a 15 hh–16 hh horse, weighs about 4 kg. Its surface area is approximately 14 000 cm^2 and it is about 1 mm thick. The foal's birth weight is directly proportional to the surface area of the placenta, as a small placenta limits the amount of nutrients which can pass to the fetus. In extreme cases abortion can be caused if the size of the placenta is restricted for some reason such as, uterine infection, old age and twins.

1.4.3.1 Twins

Twinning is an increasing problem in stud management, especially in intensively bred horses such as the thoroughbred. The incidence of twin ovulations, which can result in twin pregnancies in the thoroughbred is 20–25%. Nature does naturally reduce many of these pregnancies to a single (up to 70%). However, if twins do develop to the

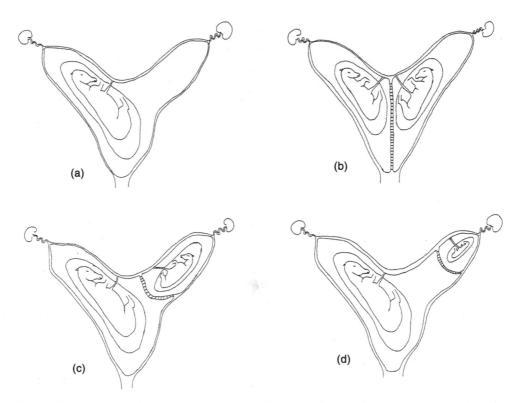

Figure 1.30 Placental arrangements in the single equine fetus and twin pregnancies (a) single, (b) equal split (50%:50%), (c) unequal split (60%:40%), (d) unequal split (80%:20%). © CABI.

placenta stage, the area of the uterus available for each placenta is restricted by the presence of the other fetus. Occasionally the division of the uterine surface between each twin is equal (Figure 1.30 (b)), this is the only chance that both twins may survive but their birth weights will be reduced. Normally the division is unequal, in which case the smaller twin may cause the whole pregnancy to abort (Figure 1.30 (c)) or, if the pregnancy is not well advanced, it (i.e. the smaller twin) may die and become mummified (Figure 1.30 (d)). If mummification occurs the pregnancy may continue but as the placenta of the larger surviving fetus is restricted (Figure 1.31) a smaller than expected single foal will be born.

1.5 LACTATION

At first it might be thought that lactation in the mare is not particularly important, especially when compared to the dairy cow. However,

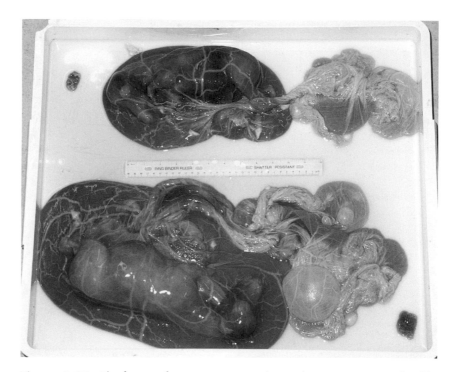

Figure 1.31   The fetuses of a twin pregnancy dissected out post mortem. The different size of the twins is evident and is the result of placental restriction of the smaller twin. If left to go to term the smaller twin would eventually have died and may have caused the abortion of the whole pregnancy.

its importance in the mare must not be underestimated as lactation has a direct effect on the growth and development of the foal. An understanding of lactation is important if this natural food is to be used to maximum advantage by providing the best start in life for the foal.

1.5.1 Anatomy of the mammary gland

Milk is produced in the udder or mammary gland. Different mammals have a different number of mammary glands situated along the abdomen either side of the mid-line in pairs; pigs have up to 10 pairs, whereas primates have only one pair. The mare has two pairs of glands (four in total) situated between the hind legs (the inguinal region), protected by a layer of skin and hair although the teat area is hairless and particularly sensitive. The whole mammary gland is supported by, and attached to the body of the mare, by sheets of ligament (Figure 1.32).

In most mammals, each gland has its own teat, so in the mare you would expect there to be four, however, the mare is relatively unique

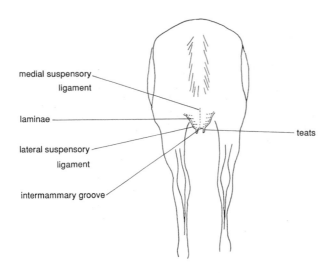

medial suspensory ligament

laminae

teats

lateral suspensory ligament

intermammary groove

Figure 1.32 A rear view of the mare's udder, illustrating the suspensory ligaments of the mammary gland. © CABI.

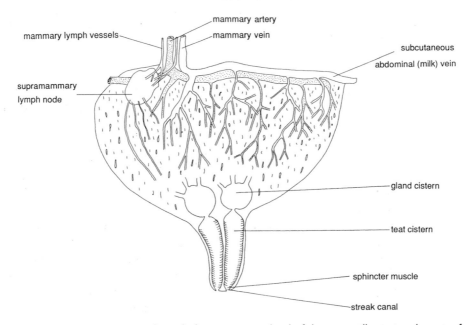

mammary lymph vessels

mammary artery

mammary vein

subcutaneous abdominal (milk) vein

supramammary lymph node

gland cistern

teat cistern

sphincter muscle

streak canal

Figure 1.33 A cross-section through the mammary gland of the mare, illustrating the exit of two quarters via a single teat. © CABI.

in that each pair of glands, either side of the mid-line, has a single teat, and so in fact the mare has only two teats (Figure 1.33).

The milk-producing tissue within the mammary gland is made up of millions of alveoli and interconnecting ducts. The alveoli, the milk-secreting structures, are lined with lactating cells, which surround a

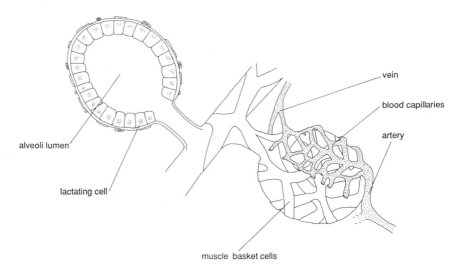

Figure 1.34 The mammalian alveolus. On the left, a cross-section illustrating the lactating cells surrounding the alveolar lumen, which is continuous with the mammary gland duct system. On the right, an alveolus illustrating the muscle cells and blood supply. © CABI.

central cavity or lumen (Figure 1.34), which is continuous with the ducts of the gland. Milk is secreted by the lactating cells into the lumen and on to the teats for storage ready for the foal at suckling. Each alveolus is surrounded by muscle cells and blood capillaries which supply them with nutrients and the components required for milk.

These alveoli are grouped together and are connected via a network of ducts which eventually join and empty into the gland cistern – the milk storage area above each teat (Figure 1.33). This arrangement may be compared with a bunch of grapes, the grapes being the alveoli and the stalks the interconnecting ducts (Figure 1.34). At the end of each teat is a tight sphincter muscle which prevents the leakage of milk between sucklings.

1.5.2 Lactation curve

Figure 1.35 illustrates the lactation curve for a typical mare, that is, the amount of milk produced at different times after the birth of her foal. This lactation curve can be altered quite significantly by the way we manage the mare and her foal in early life.

Milk production increases over the first four to eight weeks of lactation until a peak is reached of around 10–18 litres/day in thoroughbreds or 8–12 litres/day in ponies. This is compared to up to 50

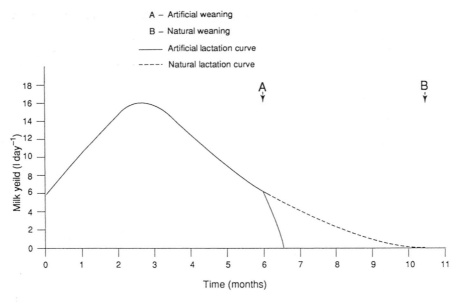

Figure 1.35 The average lactation curve for a mare, illustrating the natural lactation curve as well as the effect of weaning at six months. © CABI.

litres/day produced by a good dairy cow. After eight weeks or so the foal normally begins to get nutrients from sources other than milk, such as grass and hay, or creep feed in managed foals. As the foal obtains more food elsewhere, the demand for milk reduces and so milk production declines. In managed mares and foals, we manipulate the shape of the lactation curve by providing the foal with supplementary food in the form of creep feed. Creep feed is fed at different times by different systems. If creep feed is fed from about one week of age the foal starts to get nutrients elsewhere more quickly and so relies less on its dam's milk. In this case maximum milk yield occurs earlier and the total amount of milk produced is reduced to match the demands of the foal. If creep feed is not fed until week six or so, then the foal will rely on its dam's milk for longer, its demands will be greater, so maximum lactation yield occurs later and the total amount of milk produced is greater. In wild ponies lactation occurs for ten to eleven months, the mare normally dries off and rejects the foal a few weeks before the next foal is due to be born. This gives the mammary gland about four weeks to recover and to start to build up colostrum in readiness for the new foal. If the mare is not in foal again the foal may still suckle up to eighteen months of age. In managed systems most foals are weaned at six months and so milk production drops off dramatically at this time (Section 8.4, p. 193).

Table 1.3 The average composition of mare's milk during the main part of lactation.

Component	Percentage (%)
Water	89.0
Casein protein	1.4
Whey protein	1.3
Lactose	6.1
Fat	1.6
Ash (minerals, vitamins etc.)	0.6
Total	100.0

The total milk yield in the average thoroughbred mare is 2000–3000 litres, or 2–3 litres/100 kg body weight per day in larger horses and 5 litres/100 kg body weight/day in ponies. This compares to a total lactation milk yield in the average dairy cow of 7000 litres.

1.5.3 Milk quality

Not only does milk production vary according to the stage within the lactation curve, but so does the quality. In general, the quality reflects the needs of the foal and provides energy and the requirements for growth and development (Table 1.3). One of the major changes in milk composition is the production of colostrum in very late pregnancy and for the first twelve hours after birth. From twelve hours after birth onwards normal milk is then produced.

1.5.3.1 Colostrum

Colostrum, sometimes termed the first milk, contains a high concentration of proteins. These proteins are antibodies, and as a result the initial protein concentration of milk is 13.5%, compared with 2.7% during main lactation. Within twelve hours these high protein levels decline as antibodies are no longer present. The digestive system of the foal is only able to absorb complete protein molecules, such as antibodies, for the first twenty-four hours of life. It is essential, therefore, that a newborn foal receives its colostrum well within twenty-four hours of birth, after this time it cannot take advantage of any antibodies in the colostrum (Section 7.2.7.1, p. 166).

1.5.4 Milk synthesis and secretion

Milk is synthesised (made) in the lactating cells lining each alveoli (Figure 1.34). The precursors (building blocks) of milk are obtained from the blood system supplying the mammary gland. These components cross the cell membrane into the lactating cells where milk protein, fat and lactose are then built up from the amino acids, glycerol, free fatty acids and glucose in the blood. Once the components of milk have been built up they pass into the lumen of the alveoli and on through the ducts to the gland cistern ready for the foal. Milk contains 89% water, which also passes from the blood through the lactating cell to the lumen by the process of diffusion.

1.6 CONCLUSION

A knowledge of reproductive anatomy forms the basis for an understanding of reproductive control. This knowledge can then be used to make educated decisions about introducing or changing management practices to the benefit of horse welfare and production.

Control of Reproduction

2.1 INTRODUCTION

An understanding of how reproduction is controlled naturally is essential before any artificial manipulation of reproduction can be considered. The mare has many more stages of reproduction (oestrous cycles, pregnancy and lactation) than the stallion and as a result most research to date has been directed towards the mare. However, the stallion is as important and a knowledge of the natural control of reproduction in the stallion is necessary if a breeding scheme or stud is to be successful.

2.2 THE MARE

In her natural state the mare is a seasonal breeder, that is, she will only breed or show sexual activity during the spring, summer and autumn, this is termed the breeding season. Winter is the non-breeding season or anoestrus. On average the breeding season lasts from April until October in the northern hemisphere and October to May in the southern hemisphere, although this can vary with breed of mare. In general 'cold-blooded' horses, such as ponies and the larger, heavier breeds tend to show shorter seasons than the finer, more 'hot-blooded' types, e.g. the thoroughbred. Regardless of the length of her breeding season the mare shows a regular series of oestrous cycles throughout her season.

2.2.1 The oestrous cycle

The oestrous cycle of the mare is divided into a period of sexual interest (oestrus or heat, 4–5 days) followed by a period of disinterest (dioestrus, 16–17 days). These cycles start at puberty (from between 10–24 months of age) and each one lasts 21 days. Each cycle is a pattern of changes in: hormone secretion; the appearance of the reproductive tract and behaviour. Ovulation occurs during oestrus, normally 24–36 hours before the end of the cycle and this is known as Day 0. The remainder of the cycle is then divided into Days 1–21 until ovulation reoccurs. The cycle is often also divided into two phases called the luteal (under the control of the corpus luteum) and follicular (follicle development) phases.

The mare is unusual among mammals in showing her first oestrus very soon after foaling, often within 4–10 days; this oestrus is known as the foal heat. After the foal heat the mare should show her regular 21-day cycle, but it is worth noting that the cycles can be irregular for a couple of cycles.

2.2.1.1 Control of the natural cycle

The oestrous cycle can be more easily understood if it is looked at under three headings: changes in hormone levels, changes in the reproductive tract and changes to the mare's behaviour – it must be remembered however that all three areas are closely interrelated.

2.2.1.1.1 Changes in hormone secretion within the oestrous cycle

The hormones which control the oestrous cycle are secreted by the hypothalamus and the pituitary gland (in the brain) as well as by the ovaries and uterus. The interaction between the hypothalamus, pituitary gland and ovaries form the hypothalamic-pituitary-gonadal (ovarian) axis and it is this axis which controls the sexual activity of the mare (Figure 2.1).

Activity within this axis is determined by day length (known as photoperiod) with environmental temperature and nutrition having a lesser effect. Information on day length is received by the mare's eye and passed to the pineal gland in the brain, which in turn passes the 'message' on to the hypothalamus using the hormone melatonin, which is only produced during the hours of darkness. So when day length is short and the night is long, i.e. in winter, melatonin secretion is high. Melatonin acts on the hypothalamus preventing it, and hence the hypothalamic-pituitary-ovarian axis, from functioning. When the day length increases the level of melatonin decreases, and the axis begins to function and secretes hormones which affect the ovary. During spring, summer and autumn, when day-length is long and melatonin levels lower, the hypothalamus produces a hormone called gonadotropin-releasing hormone (GnRH), which passes directly to the pituitary via specialised connecting vessels. When the GnRH reaches the anterior pituitary it causes follicle-stimulating hormone (FSH) and luteinising hormone (LH) to be produced. These hormones then pass

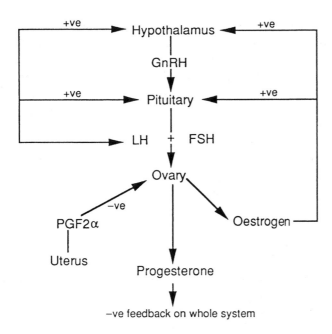

Figure 2.1 The hypothalamic–pituitary–gonadal (ovarian) axis which controls reproductive activity in the mare (−ve and +ve denotes negative and positive feedback respectively). © CABI.

into the general blood system and on to the ovaries. The level of hormones circulating within the body can be measured in blood plasma.

Follicle-stimulating hormone, or FSH, as its name suggests, is responsible for follicle development. It is passed into the blood system of the mare and appears as two peaks, one at Day 9–12 of the cycle, the smaller of the two peaks, and one at ovulation (Figure 2.2). In the mare, the follicles develop for a period of 21 days, they are then ready for ovulation to take place. Follicles start to develop at Day 0 when the last ovulation occurred; the smaller FSH peak, Day 9–12, gives a boost to this development, which is then completed by the larger FSH peak at ovulation. This usually results in one follicle being ready for ovulation.

As the follicles develop they secrete oestrogen which is released into the main blood system around the time of ovulation and passes to the brain and central nervous system (CNS) causing oestrous behaviour (heat) (Section 2.2.1.1.3). Oestrous behaviour occurs around the time of ovulation and causes the mare to accept the attentions of the stallion and allows him to mate her. The bigger the follicles the greater the amount of oestrogen they produce and maximum levels are seen 24–48 hours before ovulation (Figure 2.2). This ensures that the mare is mated just before ovulation, allowing time for the sperm to travel through the mare's tract to meet the ovum. FSH and oestrogen levels both reach a peak within oestrus, ensuring that maximum follicular development (in readiness for ovulation) and oestrus occur together (are synchronised). The 'messenger' which causes ovulation is LH, which like FSH, is secreted by the anterior pituitary gland. LH levels also rise to a peak at oestrus (Figure 2.2) and so are at a maximum at the same time as FSH and oestrogen. All this ensures that the signal for ovulation occurs when follicles are at their largest and ready to ovulate and when the mare is showing oestrous behaviour.

Once ovulation has occurred and the ova and follicular fluid, which made up the follicle, are released into the fallopian tube, the remains of the follicle collapses. Blood capillaries, which used to feed the follicle, then bleed into the cavity where the previous follicle was, forming a blood clot which is called the corpus luteum (CL). The CL secretes progesterone. Progesterone levels, therefore, rise after ovulation (Figure 2.2) and stay high for many months in the pregnant mare or until Day 14–16 of the oestrous cycle in the non-pregnant mare. If there is no pregnancy, levels of progesterone drop dramatically 4–5 days before the next ovulation. This drop in level is essential as progesterone inhibits the release of LH and reduces the secretion of FSH, so preventing ovarian activity (as ovulation is not required during pregnancy). Oestrus cannot occur until progesterone levels have fallen. Hence if the mare is not pregnant, in order for her to ovulate and show oestrus again in 21 days, progesterone levels must fall. The

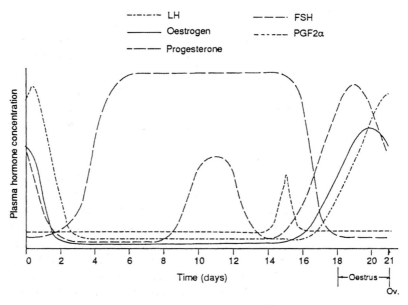

Figure 2.2 The major hormone changes within the oestrous cycle of the mare. ©
CABI.

hormone prostaglandin F2α (PGF2α) produced by the uterus is responsible for this as its role is to destroy the progesterone-producing CL.

If no pregnancy is detected by 14–16 days after the last ovulation, the mare's hormone system automatically assumes that she is not pregnant. As a result PGF2α is secreted by the uterus into the blood system and on to the ovary where it causes the destruction of the CL. The resulting drop in progesterone levels, removes any effect on LH and FSH release, and so allows these hormones to rise ready to drive the next ovulation.

2.2.1.1.2 Changes in the reproductive tract of the mare within the oestrous cycle

As well as changes in hormone levels in the 21-day cycle, changes also occur in the mare's reproductive tract. It is important to remember that these changes are driven by the changing hormone levels. High progesterone and low oestrogen levels (during dioestrus) cause secretions produced by the uterus to become thicker and also increases the thickness of the uterine wall as the endometrium (the mucous membrane lining the uterus) grows and develops. All these changes are in preparation for a potential pregnancy. If no pregnancy is present oestrus will recur, at which time progesterone levels are low and oestrogen levels are high, resulting in the above situation being reversed – the uterine wall reduces in thickness and the secretions in the uterus increase and become more fluid.

The cervix also changes with the cycle. If viewed with a vaginascope during dioestrus it appears white, firm and dry, providing an effective tight seal against bacteria. During oestrus the cervix relaxes (termed flowering) and appears moist and red, this opens the cervical seal to make mating easier but also puts the mare at risk of infection. High oestrogen levels at this point in the cycle increase the ability of the reproductive tract to fight infection, so helping to counteract this risk.

2.2.1.1.3 Changes in behaviour within the oestrous cycle

Changes in hormone levels during the oestrous cycle of the mare control her behaviour as well as the reproductive tract, determining whether the mare shows interest in the stallion (oestrus), or is hostile to him (dioestrus). The two major hormones involved are oestrogen and progesterone. High oestrogen and low progesterone levels stimulate the brain and CNS and cause oestrous behaviour. There are many variations in the exact behaviour a mare will show when she is in oestrous (Figure 2.3), this is discussed in more detail in Section 4.2.2.1, p. 81. However, a mare's general behaviour while in oestrus is:

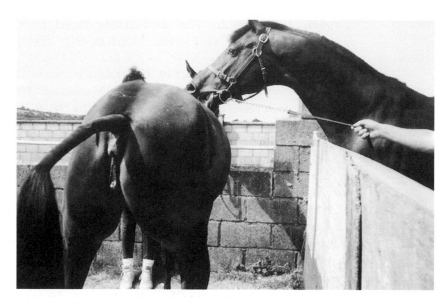

Figure 2.3   A mare showing typical signs of oestrus, standing still in the presence of the stallion and exposing her clitoris (lower part of the vulva), an event known as 'winking'. © CABI.

- docility
- characteristic urination stance
- lengthening and opening of the vulva to expose the clitoris (known as winking)
- tail raised
- urine bright yellow with a characteristic odour
- acceptance of the stallion's advances

Typical behaviour of the mare in dioestrus is:

- hostility
- rejection of stallion's advances

2.2.1.2 Artificial manipulation of the oestrous cycle

The majority of horse matings today are controlled by man (Section 4.2.2, p. 80), largely to ensure that the mare is mated at the best time to ensure fertilisation. Properly timed it can take just one mating per foal, and if this can be achieved then many more mares can be covered by a stallion during a breeding season and his owner can therefore maximise any financial return. There are two main reasons for manipulating reproduction: to advance the breeding season so that matings can occur earlier in the year or dictate the time of oestrus and ovulation within that season.

2.2.1.2.1 Advancing the breeding season

The horse is a long-day breeder, breeding from spring to autumn (Section 2.2.1.1.1, p. 38). The thoroughbred industry, and increasingly other breed societies, registers the birth of all foals on the 1 January (northern hemisphere) or 1 July (southern hemisphere) each year, regardless of their actual birth date. In the northern hemisphere, in order to have the maximum advantage in racing, thoroughbred foals should be born as soon as possible after 1 January. As the mare has an eleven-month pregnancy, mares need to be covered at the beginning of February. The artificial covering season in thoroughbreds in the northern hemisphere runs from 15 February to 1 July and in the southern hemisphere from 15 August to 31 December. Other breed societies have similar artificial breeding seasons.

The problem with these artificial breeding seasons is that they do not correspond to the natural one. The mare's breeding season needs to be brought forward artificially to ensure that the mare shows oestrus and ovulation during what would normally be her non-breeding season. There are several ways in which this can be achieved, including the use of light and hormone treatment, or a combination of the two.

2.2.1.2.1.1 Light treatment

In a group of mares housed over the winter normally only 10% will naturally show oestrus and ovulation during the non-breeding season. This figure is much lower for semi-wild ponies and horses which are wintered out. The aim with any treatment is to increase this from 10% to 100%. One of the main triggers for the start of the breeding season in spring is increasing day length (Section 2.2.1.1.1, p. 38). Manipulating day length using electric lights combined with improved nutrition and an increase in environmental temperature will increase the number of mares in oestrus during the non-breeding season.

Treatment of mares with light to advance the breeding season is common practice in many studs and was first reported in the 1940s. Mares need to experience 16 hours of light and 8 hours of dark. Light can be provided by a 200-watt light bulb, or equivalent, in a $4\,m^2$ loose-box. Light treatment can be started at any time from November onwards in the northern hemisphere and it can be introduced either suddenly or gradually. Starting treatment any earlier than November does not work as well as the mare must have experienced a reduction in day length first, similar to that of autumn. If light treatment is started in early December, the first sign that the treatment is working is that the mare will lose her coat within four weeks, and this is then followed by ovarian activity two to four weeks later. Light treatment from early December is often chosen as it results in ovarian activity during late January and early February ready for the beginning of the thoroughbred breeding season on 15 February.

The effect of increasing day length can be maximised by increasing environmental temperature and improving nutrition, both of which are also naturally associated with spring. However, temperature and nutrition have much less of an effect on oestrus than light and due to the extra costs it is often not worth doing more than rugging mares up and increasing the concentrate proportion in the diet.

Although light treatment is very successful in advancing the season, there is a lot of variability as to exactly when a mare will ovulate. In an attempt to reduce this variation, hormone treatment is sometimes used.

2.2.1.2.1.2 Hormone treatment

The use of hormones alone to induce oestrous activity in the non-breeding season of the mare is not particularly successful. It appears that the ovary of the mare during the non-breeding season is relatively insensitive to the artificial introduction of hormones (through hormone injection or treatment); a long period of treatment is required if any effect is to be seen. However, if the mare is in the transition period, that is, she is beginning to come out of the non-breeding season or dioestrus, and ovarian activity is just starting in the build-up to the breeding season, hormone treatment can work well, encouraging her to cycle early and allowing oestrus and ovulation to be timed more accurately.

2.2.1.2.1.3 Combination treatments

Many studs use of a combination of lights and hormones in the artificial manipulation of the breeding season of the mare. Light is used to advance mares into the transition period and hormones are then used to time more precisely oestrus and ovulation. The most commonly used method is a combination of light plus progesterone. Table 2.1 gives an example as to how these may be timed in practice. The exact timing of the progesterone treatment can be varied depending on when covering is planned and when light treatment is started.

Progesterone is commonly used in the management of breeding mares. Traditionally it is given either in the feed (orally, such as Regumate®) or by intramuscular injection. More recently it is available as a PRID (progesterone-releasing intervaginal device), CIDR (controlled internal drug-releasing device) and sponges, all of which are impregnated with progesterone and placed inside the mare's vagina for as long as treatment is required. Progesterone is released slowly and absorbed through the vaginal wall and into the blood system. PRID, CIDR and sponges are increasingly popular as they are labour saving,

Table 2.1 The advancement of oestrus and ovulation in the mare using light treatment and progesterone supplementation (N.B. considerable variation in individual mare's response may be observed).

Time (typical dates)	Drug to be administered /event
Day 0 (15 December)	Light treatment commences (16 hours light: 8 hours dark)
Day 28 (12 January)	Coat loss in mare may be apparent
Day 42 (26 January)	Ovarian activity may be apparent
Day 43 (27 January)	Progesterone treatment starts
Day 55 (8 February)	Progesterone treatment stops (plus possible PGF2α injection)
Day 60+ (13 February)	Oestrus commences
Day 62+ (15 February)	Ovulation may occur – covering/AI

only having to be inserted and removed at the end of treatment. They also guarantee that a standard dose is given. In common with these, progesterone injection also guarantees that each mare receives her correct dose. However, the injection method is more expensive, especially if a veterinary surgeon is required to administer injections (a legal requirement in UK). Putting progestagen in the feed (Regumate®) has the advantage that no vet is required, but mares have to be fed individually and some mares may refuse to eat the feed in which it is mixed, so there is no guarantee the mare has had the correct dose.

As an alternative to progesterone a series of two or three PGF2α injections 48 hours apart can be used to 'kick start' the cycle. However, it is more normally administered as a single injection as illustrated in Table 2.1 when progesterone treatment is stopped. Even when using a combination of light and hormones there is still some variation in the timing of oestrus and ovulation. However, most mares will show oestrus within 5–10 days and ovulate within 7–14 days of the end of progesterone treatment.

2.2.1.2.2 Synchronisation and timing of oestrus

In addition to manipulating the timing of oestrus, advancing the breeding season makes mare management easier. In many countries, for example South America and the United States, mares roam in large herds over vast areas of land. Such systems require handling to be kept to a minimum. It is ideal, therefore, if all mares can be treated in batches from conception to birth and foal rearing. To do this, batches of mares have to be mated at the same time, that is, have their oestrous cycles synchronised.

The same treatment can also be used in mares for which teasing, rectal palpation or scanning is inconvenient or for artificial insemination and embryo transfer.

Table 2.2 The timing of oestrus and ovulation in the mare using progesterone supplementation, with suggested timings for AI (N.B. considerable variation in individual mare's response may be observed).

Time	Drug to be administered/event
Day 0–14	Progesterone supplementation (inter-vaginal sponges or PRID, intramuscular (i.m.) injection or oral administration)
Day 17 onwards	Oestrus may start
Day 20 onwards	Ovulation may occur – covering/AI

The methods used to time oestrus and ovulation are very similar to those used to advance the breeding season and are also based upon the hormones naturally produced during the oestrous cycle. There are two ways of timing oestrus, to lengthen the natural luteal phase (when the CL is dominant) and then determine its ending (progesterone treatment with a timed end to treatment); or to time the end of the natural luteal phase (i.e. destroy the CL at a specific time using PGF2α) (Figure 2.4).

Progesterone treatment, by any of the various methods, gives the mare an artificially long luteal phase (artificial CL). Stopping progesterone treatment will end this luteal phase and can be timed so that the date of oestrus and ovulation is predicted (Figure 2.4 (b)). The end of the artificial luteal phase, like the natural one, induces the changes in hormones responsible for oestrus and ovulation. Within two to three days of the start of progesterone treatment a mare will stop all oestrous activity, she will remain like this until the end of treatment. Indeed competition mares are often treated with progesterone for long periods of time, to stop oestrous behaviour especially when competing. For synchronising or timing oestrus, progesterone is normally given for 10–15 days and then stopped, after which oestrous behaviour starts within 3–7 days and ovulation occurs at 6–10 days (Table 2.2).

PGF2α can be used to end the natural luteal phase by destroying the CL, this again allows the hormones which control oestrus and ovulation to increase (Figure 2.4 (c)). The success of PGF2α in timing oestrus in the mare is variable and depends upon the stage of the cycle. PGF2α will only work when the mare has a CL that is between Days 4 and 14 of the cycle. This is no problem if the mare's cycle is being monitored. However, the stage of cycle is not always known especially in big herds of mares, so two injections of PGF2α have to be administered 12–14 days apart to guarantee a response. Most mares will show oestrus and ovulate within 3–7 days of PGF2α treatment (second injection if two are given) (Table 2.3).

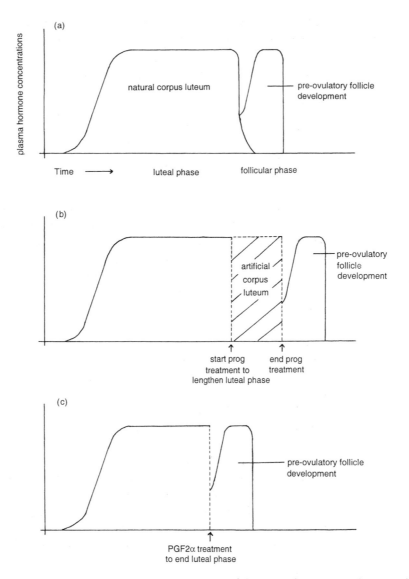

Figure 2.4 A diagram of the oestrous cycle of the mare showing: (a) the natural cycle; (b) the artificial lengthening of the luteal phase (using progesterone); and (c) the artificial shortening of it (using PGF2α). Artificial manipulation of the luteal phase is used to time oestrus.

Both progesterone and PGF2α work well alone but they still do not give an exact timing of oestrus and ovulation, so combination treatments plus additional hormones such as human chorionic gonadotropin (hCG) and gonadotropin-releasing hormone (GnRH) can be used. PGF2α can be given at the end of progesterone treatment

Table 2.3 The timing of oestrus and ovulation in the mare using a single injection of prostaglandin (N.B. considerable variation in individual mare's response may be observed).

Time	Drug to be administered/event
Day 0	Oestrus
Day 7	Prostaglandin (via intramuscular (i.m.) injection)
Day 10	Oestrus commences
Day 12	Ovulation may occur – covering/AI

(mimicking the natural PGF2α rise at the end of the cycle) and gives a more predictable timing of oestrus and ovulation. HCG is similar to LH and so causes ovulation if given to a mare with a large, mature follicle. It is sometimes used a couple of days after administration of PGF2α or after the end of progesterone treatment to encourage ovulation. Mares are often scanned regularly as they approach ovulation, hCG can then be administered as soon as a mature follicle is identified. This will cause the mare to ovulate within the next 24–48 hours, and helps to ensure that the mare is covered at the best time. Recent research has suggested that the mare develops antibodies to hCG, and therefore hCG does not work well in mares which have been treated many times before. In this case GnRH is sometimes used to encourage a quick natural release of LH that then acts in the same way as the hCG to cause ovulation (Section 2.2.1.1.1, p. 38).

A number of these hormones may be used together. In general the closer the treatment mimics the natural cycle the better the response, however any improvement in response is often not worth the extra cost and labour. In practice either progesterone, PGF2α or a combination of the two are used on most studs along with ultrasonography or rectal palpation, to accurately predict the timing of ovulation. Many of these synchronisation treatments can also be used to induce ovulation and oestrus in mares with abnormal oestrous cycles, acting to 'kick start' the system again.

2.2.2 Pregnancy (gestation)

Understanding hormone control during pregnancy is essential before problems such as abortion can be understood and appropriate treatment considered.

2.2.2.1 Natural control of pregnancy

By Day 6 the conceptus has travelled to the uterus, though no major differences in hormone levels are evident yet between pregnant and non-pregnant mares. However, by Day 15 a 'message' from the embryo has to be received by the reproductive system of the mare if it is to continue in pregnancy mode. This 'message' stops the release of PGF2α which, in the non-pregnant mare, causes the destruction of the CL. High progesterone is essential for the maintenance of pregnancy and a drop in levels will cause abortion. Initially progesterone is secreted by the ovary.

In non-pregnant mares progesterone levels drop at Day 15, whereas in pregnant mares they remain high, rising again around Day 35–45 and then remaining high throughout the rest of pregnancy. If the ovary of the pregnant mare is examined around Day 35–40 new CL-like structures (known as secondary CL) appear, these help to keep up the ovary's production of progesterone. These secondary CL, plus the first (or primary) CL, continue to secrete progesterone until about Day 150 of pregnancy although from Day 75 onwards, progesterone secretion by all the CL begins to decline. However, high progesterone levels must be maintained in order to keep the pregnancy, so at this stage the placenta begins to secrete progesterone, gradually taking over from the CL. By Day 150 progesterone comes only from the placenta, and this continues to the end of pregnancy, though after Day 240–300 levels start to decline steadily.

Around Day 40 a unique hormone appears in the mare's blood – this is equine chorionic gonadotropin (eCG) also known as pregnant mare serum gonadotropin (PMSG). This hormone is secreted by the endometrial cups (Section 1.4.3, p. 26) and can be detected in the mare's blood from Day 40 to Day 120. There are several theories regarding the role of eCG; it may prevent the mare's uterus from rejecting the conceptus, or it may cause development of the secondary CL.

Oestrogen can be detected in the pregnant mare's blood, but not until Day 40, after which levels remain high throughout the rest of pregnancy. This oestrogen comes from the ovary and is secreted by the developing follicles which go on to form the secondary CL, in a similar way to oestrogen produced by follicles before ovulation and oestrus in the normal oestrous cycle. As with progesterone the placenta gradually takes over oestrogen production, starting from Day 60–70, and continuing for the rest of pregnancy. The oestrogen secreted by the placenta is unique and different from that produced by the ovary, there are two sorts called equilin and equilenin.

2.2.2.2 Artificial manipulation of pregnancy

The artificial manipulation of pregnancy consists of shortening pregnancy (abortion) or prolonging pregnancy (preventing abortion).

Pregnancies are rarely aborted except in the case of emergencies, i.e. twins or grossly abnormal fetuses. If abortion is required PGF2α is normally given, and if used early in pregnancy a single injection is enough and can allow the mare to return to oestrus and be re-covered in time to conceive another foal that year. In order for the mare to return to oestrus on Day 21 of the cycle, i.e. as if she had never conceived in the first place, the conceptus must be aborted before Day 15 of the pregnancy. Before Day 40, the stage at which endometrial cups develop, a single injection will cause abortion and still allow the mare to return to oestrus relatively rapidly. However, abortion after Day 40 will result in a long delay in the mare's return to oestrus and the further advanced the pregnancy, the greater the dose of PGF2α that is required.

Attempts have been made, using progesterone, to keep pregnancies in mares which have a history of abortion or are showing signs that they may abort, particularly before Day 40. Indeed some studs routinely treat their mares with progesterone for the first 100 days of pregnancy as a safety measure. From Day 100 onwards placental progesterone alone should be sufficient to maintain the pregnancy. Though progesterone treatment is often used there is no scientific evidence to support that it works.

2.2.3 Parturition (birth)

Pregnancy (gestation) in the mare lasts approximately eleven months (310–374 days). The exact length, however, varies with breed; ponies tend to foal two weeks before thoroughbred mares (320 days compared to 335 days). Mares mated early in the season tend to have longer pregnancies than those mated later on and colt foals are born about three days later than filly foals. The mare herself may also affect the precise hour of foaling most preferring to foal at night in a quiet environment.

2.2.3.1 Natural control of parturition

Parturition (birth) involves the expulsion of the fetus, placenta, and associated fluids and is caused by muscle activity within the uterus and surrounding structures (Section 6.3, p. 140). It is known that fetal development affects when parturition occurs. As pregnancy comes to an end the fetus is growing rapidly and making increasing demands on the placenta (in terms of nutrition plus oxygen uptake and carbon dioxide removal) in order to survive and continue to grow. The placenta reaches a stage when it can no longer supply what the fetus demands and so the fetus becomes stressed. In addition, as the foal grows it becomes restricted within the uterus, it can no longer move as freely within the uterus, further increasing stress.

These stresses eventually drive the hormone changes that result in parturition.

Uterine muscle activity is inhibited (prevented) by high progesterone levels. At parturition progesterone levels fall and this allows muscle activity to occur. Uterine muscle contraction is then driven by sharp increases in levels of prostaglandin F2α (PGF2α) and another hormone called oxytocin just before parturition. Both PGF2α and oxytocin cause the cervix to dilate and drive strong uterine muscle contractions.

Parturition consists of three stages (Section 6.3, p. 140); stage 1, positioning of the foal within the uterus, which requires minimum muscle contraction; stage 2, delivery of the foal, which requires maximum muscle contraction; and stage 3, delivery of the placenta, which, like stage 1, requires minimum muscle contraction. Levels of PGF2α rise first and this hormone is involved in stages 1 and 2, oxytocin levels rise slightly later and is involved in stages 2 and 3.

2.2.3.2 *Artificial manipulation of parturition*

Artificial manipulation of parturition is not practiced regularly. Most intervention is limited to the induction of parturition, which is very similar to induced abortion (Section 2.2.2.2, p. 49). In order for parturition to be induced successfully it is very important that the fetus is mature enough to survive outside the uterus. As the length of pregnancy varies greatly in the mare this can be difficult to assess. The most practical method is to analyse secretions from the mammary glands, in particular to ascertain levels of calcium; concentrations above 4 mg/ml indicate that the fetus has a good chance of surviving. In general parturition is only induced in an emergency, such as very long gestation, colic, pelvic injury, rupture, painful arthritic conditions etc. in order to try and save the mare. Oxytocin is the most common hormone used, although PGF2α may also be used. Multiple low-dose injections of the chosen hormone are the best method and allow uterine muscle contractions to gradually build up rather than inducing a sudden contraction with a single, higher dose, which runs a higher risk to mare and foal. Oxytocin is also very successfully used in cases of retained placenta (failure of stage 3).

2.3 THE STALLION

The stallion, like the mare, is in his natural state a seasonal breeder, that is, his best breeding performance is seen during the spring, summer and autumn, which is the breeding season. Maximum spermatogenesis (sperm production, measured as sperm concentration and total semen volume) and libido (sexual interest) occurs during the breeding season but given enough encouragement most stallions will mate a mare during the non-breeding season. In the stallion the non-breeding season results in a decrease in breeding performance rather than a complete stop as seen in the mare.

2.3.1 Spermatogenesis

Unlike the mare the stallion does not show cycles of sexual interest and disinterest. Spermatogenesis is a continuous process. Each individual spermatozoa undergoes 57 days' development from germ cell to mature spermatozoa. This series of events is happening to millions of developing sperm at the same time, and all are at slightly different stages along the 57-day cycle. This ensures a continual supply of fresh mature spermatozoa ready to be ejaculated and to replace any old sperm.

2.3.1.1 Natural control of spermatogenesis

As with the mare, reproductive activity starts at puberty and continues for the rest of a stallion's life, though semen quality may decline after he has reached 20 years of age. The exact timing of puberty varies with breed and development but usually occurs at 12–24 months, however full reproductive ability, that is, the ability to cover a full book of mares (50–100) is not reached until 5–6 years of age.

The reproductive activity of the stallion can be divided into hormone secretion and behavioural changes.

2.3.1.1.1 Hormone secretion
Many aspects of hormone control in the stallion are similar to those in the mare; the overall control of stallion reproduction is controlled by the hypothalamic-pituitary-gonadal axis, though in the case of the stallion the testes are the gonads (Figure 2.5).

In exactly the same way as seen in the mare, day length, nutrition and environmental temperature have an overall effect on this axis (Section 2.2.1.1.1, p. 38) however in the stallion short day length makes the axis less efficient rather than shutting it down completely. Again as seen in the mare, gonadotrophin-releasing hormone, GnRH, is produced by the hypothalamus, which causes the anterior pituitary to produce luteinising hormone, LH, and follicle-stimulating hormone, FSH. These two hormones then pass via the blood system to the testes. Within the testes there are two cell types, the Leydig cells and the Sertoli cells (Figure 1.19, p. 19). LH acts upon the Leydig cells which

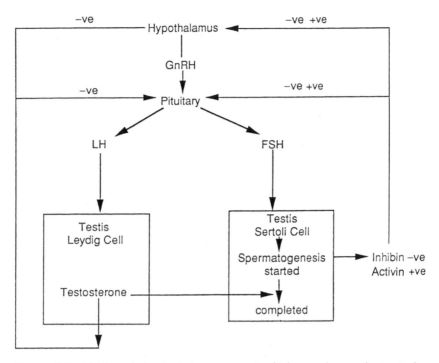

Figure 2.5 The hypothalamic-pituitary-testes axis which controls reproduction in the stallion. © CABI.

react by producing testosterone, FSH acts upon the Sertoli cells which nurse the developing spermatids. FSH drives the first stages of spermatogenesis, the final stages are driven by testosterone which is produced in the neighbouring Leydig cells. Not only does testosterone have an effect on spermatogenesis but it also plays an important role in the development of male genitalia, the descent of the testes, changes seen at puberty, the physical characteristics of the stallion, such as accelerated growth and muscle development, as well as the maintenance and function of the accessory glands. It is also responsible for male libido and sexual behaviour.

Testosterone also feeds back on the pituitary gland and hypothalamus to control the release of LH thereby controlling its own levels. High testosterone levels reduce the release of GnRH from the hypothalamus and LH from the pituitary. Testosterone, therefore acts as a brake on its own production, ensuring a steady state or level of testosterone secretion is achieved for each individual stallion. Spermatogenesis must also be kept at a steady rate. This is achieved through the interaction of two hormones called activin and inhibin, both are produced by the Sertoli cells in response to the level of sperm production. If sperm production is too low, activin is secreted which acts on the hypothalamus and pituitary driving the production of more FSH, in turn increasing sperm production. Inhibin acts in the opposite way inhibiting the release of FSH if sperm production is too great.

The testes of the stallion are unusual in secreting high levels of oestrogen; the presence of oestrogen is one of the tests to determine whether a stallion has been successfully gelded or is a cryptorchid (Section 1.3.4, p. 16).

2.3.1.1.2 Behavioural changes

Testosterone drives male behaviour, both general stallion behaviour and the behaviour associated with mating. There is a much variation between individuals, but in general the sight of a mare drives increased testosterone secretion causing typical stallion mating behaviour. The stallion will fix his eyes upon the mare, arch his neck, stamp or paw the ground and generally pull himself up to his full height. He will often show the characteristic flehmen response of drawing back his top lip as if tasting the air and will 'roar' (Figure 2.6). This behaviour ends in mounting, mating and ejaculation and is directly affected by testosterone levels. At the beginning and the end of the breeding season when testosterone levels are lower, the stallion takes much longer to react to a mare and the number of mounts per ejaculate is greater.

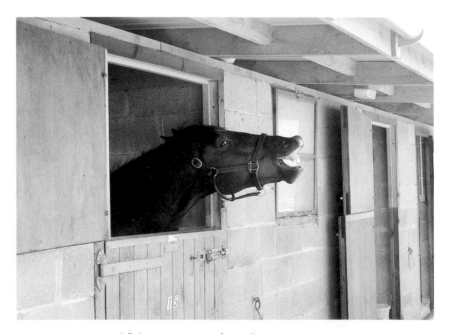

Figure 2.6 Typical flehmen response of a stallion near a mare in oestrus.

2.3.1.2 *Artificial control of spermatogenesis*

Unlike the mare, if given enough encouragement most stallions will mate during the non-breeding season. In many studs the mare's breeding season is advanced artificially (Section 2.2.1.2.1, p. 43). So that stallions can cover these mares efficiently they can also have their seasons brought forward using artificial light, (16 hours light: 8 hours dark) from mid-December onwards, this increases a stallion's libido and semen quality. Therefore, in some studs lights in the stallion boxes are put on the same timeswitch as those in the mare's boxes and their concentrate feed increased at about the same time.

2.4 CONCLUSION

It is important to understand how reproduction is controlled naturally before any consideration can be given to managing it artificially or to manipulating reproductive activity. The cyclical nature of the reproductive activity of the mare means that she is often the limiting factor in this process and so more money and time is invested in timing oestrus and ovulation in the mare than spermatogenesis in the stallion.

Selecting and Preparing the Mare and Stallion for Breeding

3.1 INTRODUCTION

Getting your mare in foal can be the most challenging and potentially most rewarding aspect of keeping a mare.

Reproductive activity in the mare starts at puberty, 10–24 months. In theory it is possible to cover a mare at this time, however it is not ideal to do so as up until she reaches her mature size (4–6 years of age) she will need to continue to grow and develop and maintain herself as well as her pregnancy. Whatever the age of your mare, it is essential that the decision to breed is taken in good time so that her suitability can be assessed and she can be prepared. The selection of a stallion and his preparation for the breeding season also needs some consideration.

3.2 SELECTING THE MARE FOR BREEDING

Many people put a lot of time and effort into selecting their mare for conformation, athletic performance etc. and then matching these to the chosen stallion's characteristics. In addition to these, selection for reproductive ability must also be considered. Failure to do so risks wasting significant amounts of money trying to get a mare in foal. By paying attention to a number of factors, many of which you can assess yourself, you can significantly increase the chances of your mare becoming pregnant. If you are the owner of a single mare you will not have a choice of mares to breed from but an understanding of what affects reproductive success will help your decision as to whether or not to breed your mare and may forewarn of problems.

There are a number of reproductive characteristics which can be assessed when considering a mare for breeding. Many of them may not exclude her from breeding but all go towards developing a picture of the mare and her likely chances of being a good broodmare.

One of the first things to consider is the mare's history. Most reputable owners will have full records of any mare and these should answer questions such as, whether her cycle is regular, she has suffered any infections, been pregnant before, and if so the number of foals, twins, abortions, problem foalings etc. In addition an answer to questions regarding usual length of her oestrous cycle, when her breeding season normally starts and finishes, whether she demonstrates oestrus better under certain circumstances, will all greatly help in her management. Information should also be obtained on vaccination and worming history, accidents, injuries, operations, whether she suffers from COPD (chronic obstructive pulmonary disease) or EIPH (exercise induced pulmonary haemorrhage), laminitis, navicular etc. as such conditions may mean she is unsuitable to breed and could be made worse by pregnancy.

It is also worth considering the age of the mare. Mares under five years will be unproven as regards breeding. Mares over twelve years, especially if not bred before, are harder to get in foal due to a higher incidence of infections and objection to the attentions of the stallion, and will also give you fewer foals in the remainder of her life than a younger mare. Therefore mares of between five and twelve years are the best, however, you may still obtain a mare outside this range at a good price which will prove very successful.

A mare's general conformation and condition are important. If a mare is over or under condition this can be corrected by good feeding and exercise but, if a mare is very thin for example, it may be a sign of another underlying problem. A mare's general conformation will be considered when selecting for performance, but as far as reproduction is concerned the mare should have a strong back and legs to enable her to carry the extra weight of pregnancy. She should also have good heart and lung room and plenty of abdominal space. The pelvic area is also important as it contains the birth canal, so this area must be checked for any injury.

Once your mare has passed these criteria you can then turn your attention to her reproductive tract, through external and internal examination. External examination may be carried out by anyone but an internal examination will require a veterinary surgeon. Perineal conformation can be assessed (Sections 1.2.2, p. 3 and 1.2.3, p. 7) and whether the mare has undergone a Caslick's vulvoplasty operation. A Caslick's operation presents problems to a broodmare as the perineal area will need to be cut and re-sutured for each mating and always for foaling. There is a limit to the number of times this operation can be performed and this in turn limits the mare's reproductive life. Ideally,

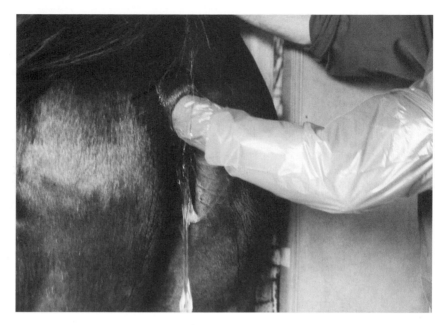

Figure 3.1 Rectal palpation in the mare allows the reproductive tract to be felt through the relatively thin rectum wall. © CABI.

such mares should be avoided. The mammary gland should be inspected for missing teats and obvious areas of damage or injury.

Internal examination involves more complicated procedures and must be carried out by a veterinary surgeon, it can, therefore, be an expensive exercise but worth it if the mare is valuable. There are a number of techniques which are used to view, or get an impression of the internal parts of the tract; these include rectal palpation, vaginascopy, ultrasonic scanning and endoscopy.

Rectal palpation can be used to give a tactile impression of the reproductive tract. A lubricated arm is inserted into the rectum and the reproductive tract felt through the thin but delicate rectum wall (Figures 3.1 and 3.2). The uterus and ovaries can be felt in turn and their texture and structures noted. As well as the tone, size and texture of the reproductive tract, the presence of cysts, tumours, stretched broad ligaments, lacerations, endometritis, scars and delayed uterine involution (failure of the uterus to return to normal size after parturition, Section 6.4.3.9, p. 159) may also be checked for.

Vaginascopy may be used to give a real image of the vagina and cervix. There are many types of vaginascope but generally they consist of a tube, with a light source at one end, which is inserted into the vagina and illuminates the internal surface of the vagina and cervix

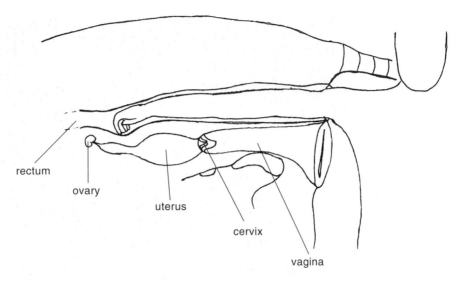

rectum

ovary

uterus

cervix

vagina

Figure 3.2 Rectal palpation in the mare. © CABI.

(Figures 3.3, 3.4 and 3.5). The vaginascope allows the vagina to be viewed directly to assess colour, lacerations, adhesions, tumours etc. The cervix can also be viewed and its appearance should match the stage of the cycle that the mare is in (Section 2.2.1.1.2, p. 41).

The endoscope, a development of the vaginascope, can be used to view through the cervix, higher up the tract, giving a real image of structures. It consists of a series of flexible carbon fibre filaments with a light source and camera attached to one end. One set of carbon fibres allows light from an external light source to pass down the endoscope, the other set transmits the image back to a camera or TV monitor (Figure 3.6). The endoscope allows the colour of the uterine endometrium, an important indicator of fertility, to be assessed. It should be uniformly pink with no dark patches. Uterine cysts, blood clots, scar tissue, adhesions etc. can be seen and any infections indicated by the presence of cloudy secretions.

Finally, ultrasonography gives a visual impression of the reproductive tract. This technique is also commonly used to predict ovulation in the mare (Section 4.2.2.2, p. 87). An ultrasonic scanner head is placed in the rectum of the mare and the flat surface directed towards the reproductive tract which lies below. The scanner emits high frequency sound waves which hit the reproductive tract, where they are either absorbed or 'bounced back' to the transducer. Whether they are absorbed or reflected depends on how dense (solid) the structures are that they hit. Dense structures bounce the sound waves back, fluids absorb them. Any sound waves which are 'bounced back' are

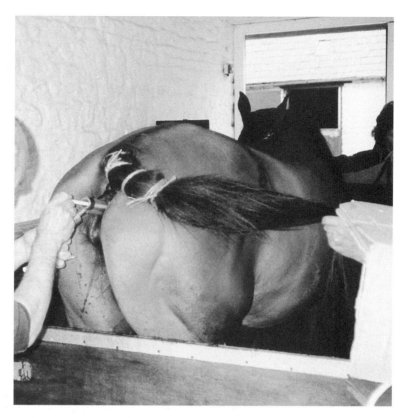

Figure 3.3   The vaginascope can be used to view the vagina and cervix and to take swabs to test for bacterial infections. © CABI.

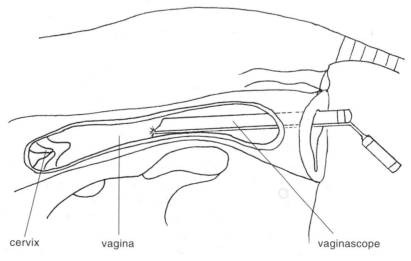

cervix   vagina   vaginascope

Figure 3.4   Vaginascopy in the mare. © CABI.

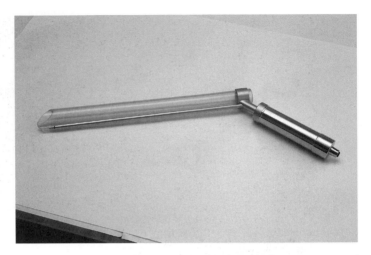

Figure 3.5   A vaginal speculum used for vaginascopy in the mare. Note the solid handle containing the batteries on the right and the small light bulb at the other end of the vaginascope (far left). © CABI.

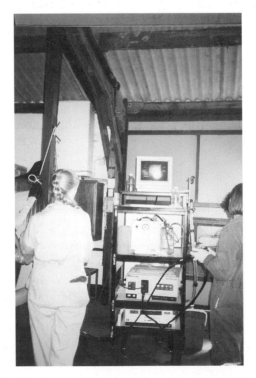

Figure 3.6   Endoscopic examination of the reproductive tract of the mare. The operator on the right controls the fibre optic camera, while the operator on the left guides the endoscope into the mare's reproductive tract. The image produced is viewed on the TV monitor. (Thoroughbred Breeders' Equine Fertility Unit, Newmarket.) © CABI.

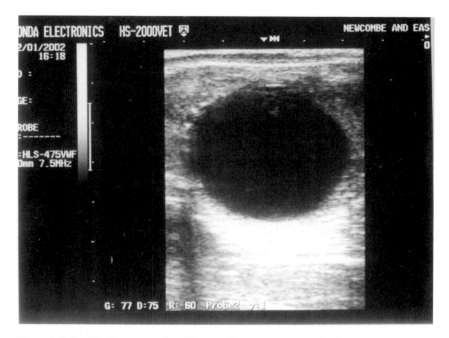

Figure 3.7 The image produced by an ultrasonic scanner of a large (4 cm diameter) follicle (large black sphere) on the ovary of the mare. Fluid areas show up as black (follicular fluid) and solid areas as white with variations in between (main ovarian tissue). Note the clear spherical shape of the follicle indicating that it is likely to ovulate in the next 48 hours. (Photograph John Newcombe.)

detected by the transducer which in turn transmits them to a monitor where they are translated into an image showing solid structures as white and fluid as black with shades of grey in between. This gives a black and white visual impression of the tract from which abnormalities such as excessive secretions, uterine cysts, tumours, etc. can be detected, along with an assessment of the state and function of the ovaries (Figures 3.7 and 3.8).

There are other techniques such as uterine biopsy, laparoscopy and laparotomy which can be used to gain further information about the mare's reproductive tract but they are rarely worth the expense and are mainly used to identify causes of infertility in very valuable mares.

The mare should also be tested for infections of the reproductive tract (Figure 3.3). The presence of infection may not preclude her from selection but will mean that she must be treated and allowed to recover before covering. Infections are a major cause of infertility and can be detected using swabs which take a sample of the secretions from the uterus, cervix, urethral opening and clitoral area (Figures 3.11 and 3.12). These are then sent away to specialised laboratories which

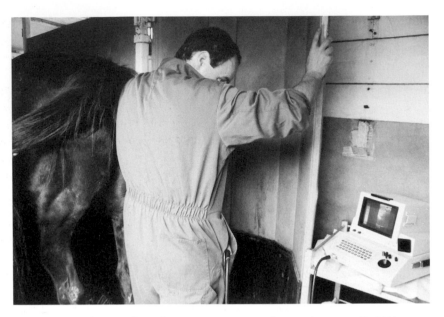

Figure 3.8 The use of an ultrasonic scanning machine in the mare. © CABI.

incubate them under different conditions (aerobic – with oxygen; anaerobic – without oxygen) and on different culture mediums. These will show the presence of any bacteria and their type, i.e. bacteria which cause venereal disease (VD) (transferred at mating). The important VD causing bacteria are: *Klebsiella pneumoniae*, *Pseudomonas aeroginosa* and *Taylorella equigenitalis* all of which may cause infertility and are passed from stallion to mare and vica versa during mating. There are a number of other bacteria such as: *Streptococcus zooepidemicus*, *Escherichia coli* and *Staphylococcus aureus* which are present in the general environment and so may also pass into the reproductive tract and cause infertility. If any of these are identified, the mare must be treated before she can be bred from (Section 3.4.1, p. 69) and her reproductive tract examined to ensure that it has not been permanently damaged by the infection. Finally, blood samples may be taken to assess red blood cell count, white blood cell count, parasite burden etc. to indicate the mare's general state of health and well-being.

3.3 SELECTING THE STALLION FOR BREEDING

As with mares people spend a lot of time and effort selecting a stallion for conformation, athletic performance etc. and matching those to the chosen mare. Reproductive ability is often overlooked. The standards of management of the stud at which the stallion stands also need to be considered. If you are choosing a stallion for purchase for breeding you will need to assess his general history, temperament and libido, age, general conformation and condition, as well as undertake external and internal examinations of his reproductive tract and a semen evaluation. However, if, as in the majority of cases, you are selecting a stallion simply to cover your mare, many of these criteria will be of limited interest to you. You will still need to be assured that fertility rates of the stallion are high so that this minimises the number of times your mare needs to be covered and, therefore, reduces both her exposure to potential infection and her keep fees.

If the stallion's fertility rates are good, then criteria such as history, age, internal and external reproductive tract examination and semen evaluation will have been met. However, you may want to consider criteria such as temperament, libido and general condition. Temperament is important in many ways and will influence ease of management, treatment of the mare and the temperament of the foal. Ideally a quiet, calm stallion, who is easy to handle should be selected. Such a stallion will be kind to mares. This is not always the case with many stallions and mares are returned to their owners with badly bitten withers and neck. Fifty per cent of the genetic make up (genotype – genetic make up of the individual) of the offspring comes from the stallion, therefore 50% of the genetic component of temperament of a foal will come from its sire. It is true to say that the environmental influence (phenotype – characteristics dictated by the way an individual is brought up and its environment) of the mare on the temperament of the foal is greater than the stallion's but there are stallions which do produce vicious, unpredictable offspring.

The overall condition of the stallion is also important as this reflects the standards of management of the stud. If he is poorly turned out, in poor condition, it is likely that your mare will return from stud in a similar condition. It is very important, therefore to visit the stud where the stallion is standing if possible and discuss their management regime. A well-run stud will give you a good impression when you visit, management will be clear, staff experienced, boxes clean and tidy, pasture in good condition and used regularly for turn out, animals will be in good condition and well kept. If your mare is to foal at the stud you should visit the foaling facilities, they should be clean, safe and roomy with a good system for 24-hour monitoring by skilled staff. The place need not be spotless but should present a good, professional image. You should talk to the stud owner about your mare and the stallion you wish to use, discuss how visiting mares are to be accommodated, and whether scanning or rectal palpation are used as well as look at the covering facilities. You also need to ask about the nomination arrangement (covering agreement), how to book your mare in and what the arrangements are for paying the covering fee etc. (Section 3.4.2, p. 71).

It is increasingly popular these days for mares not to be kept on the stallion's stud but on a neighbouring boarding yard. These boarding yards act as holding areas for mares which are to be covered by stallions in the locality. As part of the deal your mare is looked after, foaled down if required, her oestrous cycles monitored and she is taken to the stallion of your choice on the day of ovulation for covering (termed 'walking in') and then brought back to the boarding yard on the same day. She will be kept at the boarding yard for as long as you require, normally until pregnancy has been confirmed at Day 18 or 40 of the pregnancy. If you are not that happy either with your mare being kept away from home for any length of time or with the management practices of the stallion's stud and it is not too far from home, you can walk your mare in yourself on the day she is due to ovulate and take her home the same day.

There are advantages and disadvantages to all systems. If you live near the stallion then the cheapest and possibly most convenient option is to walk her in yourself. However, it may be difficult for you to determine whether your mare is in oestrus at home though ultrasonic scanning can be used (Section 4.2.2.2, p. 87). Such a system means that you have more control over the management of your mare and it avoids the upset of travel and a strange environment. If, however, you live a distance away from the stud, unless you can use artificial insemination (Section 4.3, p. 98) you will need to take your mare to board at the stud or a nearby boarding yard. Such a system may enable oestrus to be determined more accurately as all the necessary equipment and expertise is at hand. However, control over the management of your mare will lie with the stud so this needs to be considered carefully beforehand.

Ultimately the stud set up, its facilities, equipment and expertise available will reflect the type of stallion and his nomination fee. Less intensive systems such as native pony studs cannot be expected to have the level of facilities and monitoring that a thoroughbred stud has. However, the nomination and keep fees for native pony studs are much lower (typically a nomination fee of tens or hundreds of pounds) than thoroughbred studs that can stand stallions for hundreds of thousands of pounds.

3.4 PREPARING THE MARE TO GO TO STUD

When preparing a mare to be taken to stud there are a number of things which need to be considered. Careful attention should be given

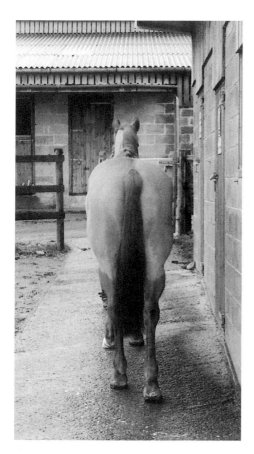

Figure 3.9 A mare in ideal body condition with a body condition score of 3. © CABI.

to the mare's body condition, which reflects her nutrition and exercise. Mares should be in good, not fat, body condition. Body condition can be scored from 0 to 5, where 5 is obese and 0 is emaciated. A condition score of 3, which is ideal for most animals, will mean that the mare is in average condition, her ribs should not be seen but can be felt and there should be no appreciable layer of fat, her neck should not have a significant crest and you should be able to see definition (outline) to the muscles of the hind quarters when she is viewed from behind (see Figures 3.9 and 3.10). The body condition score to aim for at mating is 3. In addition, it is generally believed that better conception rates in maiden and barren mares are obtained if they are on an increasing level of nutrition, in particular increasing energy, in the last four to six weeks before covering (termed flushing). This helps to 'convince' the mare that spring has arrived and improves conception rates. The best regime therefore is to ensure that the mare is in condition score 2.5 during the autumn and early winter and then four to six weeks before

Condition Score					
0	1	2	3	4	5
Pelvis/Rump/Hips					
Deep cavity under tail and either side of croup. Pelvis angular. No detectable fatty tissue between skin and bone	Pelvis and croup well defined, no fatty tissue but skin supple. Deep depression under tail	Croup well defined but some fatty tissue under skin. Pelvis easily felt, slight depression under tail	Whole pelvic region rounded not angular but easily felt. No 'gutter' along croup, skin smooth and supple	Pelvis buried in fat tissue only felt with firm pressure 'gutter' over croup	Pelvis buried in firm fatty tissue and cannot be felt. Deep 'gutter' over croup to base of dock. Skin stretched
Back/Ribs					
Processes of backbone sharp to touch. Skin drawn lightly over easily visible ribs	Ribs and backbone clearly seen, but skin is slack over bones	Backbone just covered by fat. Individual processes not visible but easily felt. Ribs just visible	Backbone and ribs covered in fat but easily felt on pressure	Backbone and ribs well covered and only felt on firm pressure. Slight 'gutter' along backbone	Backbone looks flat with deep 'gutter' along backbone. Ribs buried in fat and cannot be felt
Neck					
Ewe neck, very narrow and slack at base	Ewe neck, narrow and slack at base	Narrow but firm	No crest except for stallions	Wide and firm with folds of fatty tissue, slight crest in mares and stallions	Very wide and firm, marked crest in mares and stallions
General					
Emaciated	Thin	Fair	Good	Fat	Very Fat

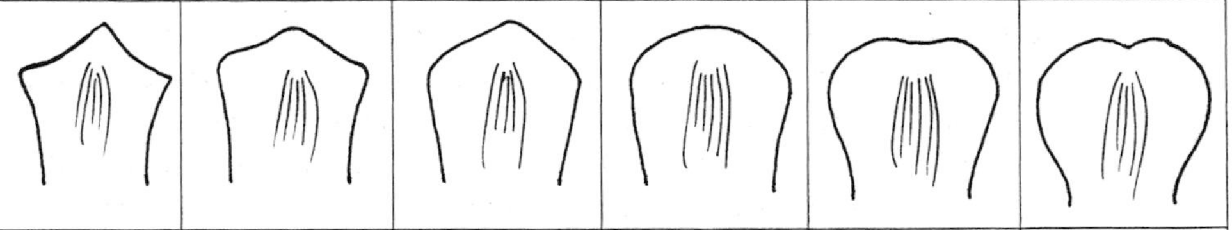

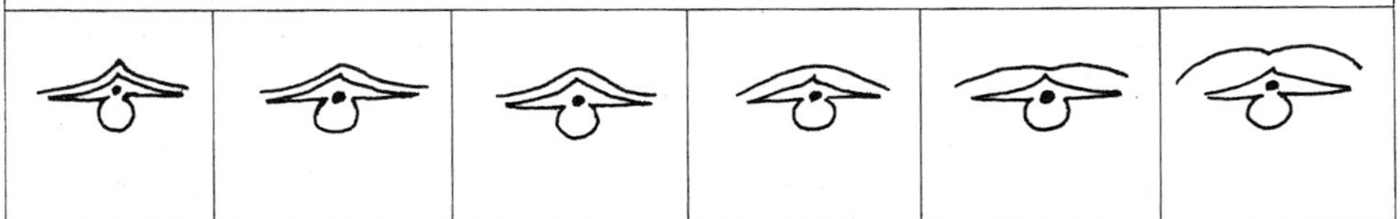

Figure 3.10 Body condition scoring in the mare.

covering increase her energy intake gradually by replacing some of her roughage with concentrates.

If your mare is young, it may also be a good idea to give her extra protein, calcium, phosphorus and vitamin A. Requirements for these are higher in young maiden mares than mature mares. It must also be remembered that if a mare is under five years of age at covering she will not have reached her mature size so her nutrition is very important since she needs nutrients to maintain both herself and the pregnancy (as with a mature mare) but also needs nutrients to continue her own growth. Her condition must be monitored carefully and her feed increased if necessary.

Exercise, which is linked to nutrition, is also important and helps to maintain body condition and prevent obesity. Gentle riding or hacking out provides a good form of exercise for barren mares during the preparation period. All mares should be turned out daily and ideally, barren mares, especially those not ridden, should live out except if the weather is really bad, providing them with *ad libitum* exercise.

Barren mares, especially maidens, should be introduced to new handling systems, buildings and surroundings associated with breeding before covering. This is of particular importance with ex-performance mares which are usually moved or sold in readiness for their new career. Making certain that mares are familiar with practices such as restraint in stocks, rectal palpation, ultrasonic scanning, teasing facilities (Section 4.2.2.1, p. 81) etc. is important in order to minimise stress. Any changes in diet must also be introduced gradually as should the introduction of new companions.

Preparation of the pregnant mare, which you plan to re-cover again after foaling, should not be forgotten, but the fact that she is pregnant means that she will not require introduction to handling systems etc. and makes flushing impossible. Exercise is still important, however, pregnant mares should not be ridden after the sixth month of pregnancy, although regular turnout is essential to maintain fitness.

3.4.1 Testing for infection

Prior to covering all mares, whether barren or pregnant, should be tested for the presence of infection in the reproductive tract. It is good practice for barren and maiden mares to have clitoral fossa swabs taken during their preparation. If these are done early enough and the result is positive then there should be enough time for treatment, recovery and retesting before mating. It is the normal practice for many studs to require mares to be swabbed and proven to be clear of infection before being accepted for covering (Figures 3.3, 3.11 and 3.12), indeed the practice is contained within the codes of practice for thoroughbred breeders. There are different recommended swabbing practices for high-risk mares (ones which have had previous contact with contagious equine metritis (CEM)) and low-risk mares (all those not classified as high-risk) as well as for those boarding at studs and walking in. It is very important that you make sure that you know and carry out the swabbing requirements before your mare goes to stud. The rules may change periodically but are published annually in the Horse Race

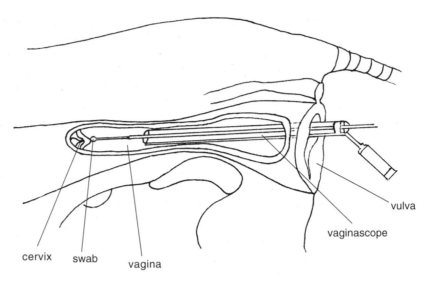

Figure 3.11   Taking a swab from the inner reproductive tract of the mare. © CABI.

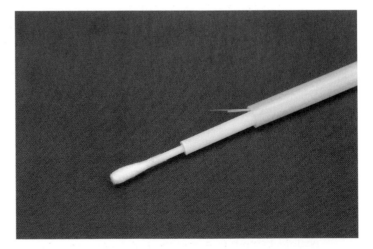

Figure 3.12   A guarded swab used to detect bacteria in the mare's reproductive tract. © CABI.

Betting Levy Board (HRBLB) codes of practice. Normally, low-risk mares must have two clean swabs, one from the clitoral fossa before the oestrus of covering, and the second from the endometrium during the oestrus of covering. High-risk mares normally need three swabs, the two which low-risk mares have, with an additional clitoral one taken before the mare arrives on the stud. All swabs must be sent to approved laboratories, the results are normally available within 48 hours and so allow enough time for mares to be covered on the oestrus of testing. Swabs are tested primarily for *Taylorella equigenitalis* the bacteria which causes CEM, but they are also tested for *Klebsiella pneumoniae* and *Pseudomonas aeruginosa*, all VD-causing bacteria. Other bacteria such as *E. coli*, *Streptococcus zooepidemicus* and *Staphylococcus aureus*, all present in the environment but which may still cause problems, may be also tested for. It must be remembered that in the UK CEM is a notifiable disease and if isolated must be reported by the testing laboratory to the divisional veterinary manager of the Department for the Environment, Food and Rural Affairs (DEFRA). The other bacterial diseases are not notifiable, but if they are identified, covering should immediately stop and advice/treatment sought. Most thoroughbred studs require a certificate for each mare indicating her previous coverings and any positive swab results (Figure 3.13). Whichever stud you are taking your mare to (except many native pony studs) it is likely that they will require paperwork to confirm that your mare is free of infection. Native pony studs do not as a rule require swabbing to take place but this should be checked during your stud selection.

In addition to bacterial infection mares may also need to be tested for viral infections. Since 1995, equine viral arteritis has also been an officially notifiable disease. It is advised that all mares have their blood tested twice, at least 14 days apart, at the beginning of the breeding season to test for antibodies. If no antibodies are present or the antibody levels are stable or declining then the mare is free of active infection and is safe to be covered. However, if increasing antibody levels are identified this means that the mare has an active infection and should not be covered. Equine herpes virus (EHV) and strangles (caused by *Streptococcus equi*) can also have disastrous consequences on breeding mares as these conditions are highly contagious and in the case of EHV cause high rates of abortion. Neither are notifiable but any mares suspected of having come into contact with EHV or strangles must be isolated and certainly not sent to stud. Veterinary advice should be sought as to whether they can be covered at all that season. The HRBLB annual codes of practice also provide advice on these conditions.

3.4.2 Nomination forms

Once a stud has been chosen and during the preparation period for your mare, a nomination form must be completed. This is a legal agreement between you and the stud owner for a nomination to a specific stallion. The exact information and agreement made varies with the stud but it will lay out the basic conditions (Figure 3.14).

CONTAGIOUS EQUINE METRITIS
AND OTHER EQUINE
BACTERIAL VENEREAL DISEASES
2004 SEASON

MARE CERTIFICATE

This certificate must be completed by the mare owner/manager and be lodged with the prospective stallion owner/manager before the mare's arrival.

Name of mare _____

Passport number (where available) _____

Name and address of owner _____

_____

Address of premises where mare currently resides _____

_____

In 2001 the above mare boarded* at _____ stud

whilst visiting _____ (stallion) result _____

In 2002 the above mare boarded* at _____ stud

whilst visiting _____ (stallion) result _____

In 2003 the above mare boarded* at _____ stud

whilst visiting _____ (stallion) result _____

Additional information including the results of positive bacteriological examinations for the CEMO, *Klebsiella pneumoniae* and *Pseudomonas aeruginosa* at any time:

_____

_____

Name (please print) _____

Signature _____ Date _____

*If no boarding stud was used, provide the name and address of the premises where the mare resided.

NB: The Thoroughbred Breeders' Association (TBA) strongly recommends that breeders consider insuring their mare against being locked-in when she visits a boarding stud or stallion stud in the UK or Ireland for the purposes of being mated. The TBA Insurance Scheme will cover the daily keep charges and veterinary treatment directly associated with the eradication of the disease. Please contact the TBA (01638 661321) for further details and premium charges.

Figure 3.13 An example of a mare certificate, required by many studs to indicate past coverings as well as any positive infections. (From the Horse Race Betting Levy Board Codes of Practice, 2004.)

BREEDING CONTRACT

STALLION ....   BOOKING FEE...........................

MARE ....   BREEDING FEE..........................

MARE AGE..   BREED......................................

COLOUR...   ID..

MARE IS: MAIDEN..............   LACTATING..................   BARREN.............

Contract:
This contract must be completed before the mare is bred. A non-refundable **Booking fee** is payable, and must be returned with this contract. Any **Boarding fee, Veterinary fee and other expenses** will be payable on receipt of an invoice or at the time the mare leaves the stud farm, whichever comes first. The **Breeding fee** will be payable at pregnancy diagnosis not later than 60 days after the last breeding.

Live foal guarantee:
The breeding is guaranteed for a foal that is born alive and stands and nurses for 24 hours. If the mare fails to produce a live foal then one return season is guaranteed providing the stallion is still available, alternatively a refund of the breeding fee will be given. Additionally the mare owner may request :
a) to substitute an acceptable mare during the next breeding season
b) a refund of the breeding fee prior to the end of the next breeding season.

Veterinarian's Certificate:
A veterinarian's health certificate including uterine culture, worming and immunization records shall be brought with the mare to the stud farm. If these documents are not presented on the mare's arrival the stud reserves the right to refuse the mare or to arrange for the resident veterinarian to take the appropriate action at the owner's expense.

Sound Condition:
The mare owner represents and warrants that each mare is in sound breeding condition and free from infection and disease. If in the opinion of the resident veterinarian any mare is not in sound breeding condition she shall not be bred.

Breeding Method:
The breeder agrees to diligently try to successfully breed the mare and shall have sole discretion in determining the best method of breeding. However, if the mare does not become pregnant the breeder shall be deemed blameless.

Breeder's Certificate:
A breeder's certificate will be issued to the mare owner after all fees and expenses have been paid and upon notification of the birth of the foal.

Registration Papers:
A copy of the mare's passport and registration papers must accompany the signed contract. The owner recorded on the registration certificate will be that recorded on the Stallion breeding report.

OWNER INFORMATION:

MARE OWNER NAME ....

ADDRESS...

....

TELEPHONE NUMBERS..

MARE OWNER SIGNATURE ....DATE........................

BREEDER/AUTHORISED AGENT NAME ....

BREEDER/AUTHORISED AGENT SIGNATURE....................................DATE........................

Figure 3.14 An example of a nomination agreement.

Some studs will require a fee or deposit to be paid on submitting the nomination form, the stud should then return acceptance as soon as possible. The terms of payment of the nomination fee depend upon the type of stud being used. A straight fee may be payable regardless of whether the mare is in foal or not, this is often the case in native pony studs and those charging a lower fee. Alternatively 'no foal, no fee October 1' terms may apply under which agreement fees are paid on covering but if the mare is proven not to be pregnant on October 1 the stud fee (excluding any keep fees) is returned. A similar arrangement is termed 'no foal, free return October 1', where instead of the fee being returned, the mare has a free cover to the same stallion or a replacement the following year. Finally for the most expensive stallions a part-payment arrangement may be made whereby 50% of the fee is due on covering and the balance paid if the mare is pregnant on October 1 or alternatively a 'live foal' arrangement may be made whereby the stud fee is returned if the mare either does not have a live foal, or has one that survives for less than 48 hours. Occasionally concessions can be given to certain mares in the form of a reduced fee to encourage good mares whose offspring will be a good advertisement for the stallion. This is most often seen with young stallions. Again it is important to check such agreements when selecting a stud.

3.4.3 General requirements

Immediately prior to sending your mare to stud she should at least have her hind shoes removed, be in good physical condition and have up-to-date tetanus and influenza vaccination certificates. She should also be wormed. Most studs will not require you to bring any tack or equipment with your mare, preferring to use their own so as to minimise the risk of losing other people's equipment. If your mare arrives at stud in good condition then it is likely that she will be returned to you in similar condition.

In order to have some control over the time of ovulation and therefore over when to cover a mare, many mares have their reproductive activity controlled with hormones (Section 2.2.1.2, p. 42). This is particularly the case with thoroughbred mares where the start of the breeding season is advanced as well as in mares covered by artificial insemination. Problem breeders may also be put on hormone programmes under veterinary advice.

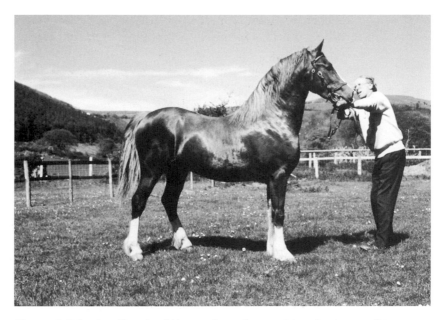

Figure 3.15   A stallion should be in a fit, not fat, condition, that is a condition score of 3 at the beginning of the breeding season. (Photograph Courtesy of Penpontpren Welsh Cob Stud, © CABI.)

3.5 PREPARING THE STALLION FOR THE BREEDING SEASON

A stallion's level of fitness is very important if he is to cope with covering a full book of mares in a season. Some thoroughbred stallions cover up to 200 mares in a short five-month season with most covers concentrated into a period of eight weeks or so. Even with fewer mares being fit, not fat, is very important. A heavy covering season places significant demands on the stallion, especially in terms of energy and he will often lose condition over the season. This loss in condition is minimised if the stallion's energy intake is increased by increasing the proportion of concentrate in his diet and if he is fit and has a body condition score of 3 at the beginning of the season (Figure 3.15). Both excess and low body weight reduce a stallion's libido. Exercise helps a stallion maintain good condition, preventing obesity and maintaining muscle tone and stamina. Stallions do have a tendency to become obese as they are often kept on their own in stables or paddocks away from each other and from mares. In natural conditions they would of course be free to exercise at will. If stallions are badly behaved it is tempting to keep them confined with only limited turnout. However this only perpetuates the problem, making misbehaviour worse due to boredom and also reduces fitness. Some stallions can be safely ridden; this provides an excellent form of exercise, as well as providing good discipline.

3.5.1 Testing for infection

The stallion, like the mare, must be free of infection before he can be allowed to breed. As with the mare, the HRBLB's annual codes of practice provide guidelines on swabbing specifically for thoroughbred stallions. These guidelines are often followed by other breed societies. Again, like mares, stallions are classified either as high-risk (those previously in contact with CEM), with the remainder classed as low-risk. All stallions should have two sets of swabs taken at an interval of no less than seven days soon after 1 January in each covering season. Swabs should be taken from the urethra, urethral fossa and the sheath of the penis. For high-risk stallions, clitoral swabs must be taken from their first four mares of the season at two days after covering. It is good practice also to swab stallions in the middle of the season or as soon as any problem is suspected. Again CEM is a notifiable disease in the UK and so must be reported to DEFRA. If any other bacteria are isolated then covering should be immediately stopped and advice/treatment sought. Once swabs have been taken and the stallion is declared clean the laboratory certificate confirming the stallion's disease-free status should be available to all mare owners.

Equine viral arteritis is also a notifiable VD in the stallion. All stallions should have their blood tested for the presence of antibodies at the beginning of the season, at least 28 days before their first mare. If no antibodies are present then the stallion is free of infection and can safely be used for covering. If antibodies are identified this may however not necessarily mean that the stallion has an active infection, veterinary advice should, therefore, be sought as to whether the stallion can be used or not.

Again in common with the mare, equine herpes virus (EHV) and strangles are potential infections. Neither is notifiable but any animals suspected of having contact with EHV or strangles must not be allowed onto a stud and if either condition is confirmed in a stallion the stud must be closed and veterinary advice sought as to whether covering can recommence that season. The HRBLB codes of practice again provide advice on these conditions.

3.5.2 General requirements

Immediately prior to the start of the season the stallion should have all shoes removed to minimise damage to mares at mounting. He should be up-to-date with his vaccinations, including influenza and tetanus, and recently wormed. Particularly in studs where the mares are walked in by their owners for covering, the stallion should be well turned out and in good condition; he should be a good advertisement for himself.

3.6 CONCLUSION

The decision to send your mare to stud requires thought and preparation if you are to maximise the chance that she will conceive safely and successfully. The preparation of a stallion is as important if he is to successfully meet the demands of a busy breeding season.

Putting Your Mare in Foal

4.1 INTRODUCTION

There are two methods by which you may choose to cover your mare: natural mating or artificial insemination (AI). Most mating management these days is driven by man's desire to control the covering process so as to minimise any risk to valuable stock and man; minimise the number of coverings per mare per foal; and ensure a specific stallion covers a specific mare.

4.2 NATURAL MATING

Natural mating is the natural physical act of covering a mare with a stallion. Within this practices vary greatly from the natural pasture breeding of wild ponies to the intensive 'in-hand' covering of very valuable stock.

4.2.1 Natural pasture breeding

In the wild, stallions run free with their harem of mares detecting whether or not they are in oestrus by examining them daily for signs of sexual acceptance. The process is leisurely and unrushed and the signals used are smell and taste rather than sight. Natural courtship may occur over several days as the mare slowly progresses from dioestrus into full oestrus, and takes place between a mare and stallion well known to each other. The mare will show that she is in full oestrus by standing still, relatively passive, curling her tail to one side, urinating, often bright yellow urine with a characteristic odour, or she may just take up the urinating stance. She will expose her clitoris (the area at the bottom of her vulva) by opening the lips of the vulva, this is termed 'winking' (Figure 2.3, p. 42). When she is fully in oestrus the stallion will mate her.

If a mare is not in oestrus she will be aggressive to the stallion who will be unable to get closer to her than the initial advance. The stallion will then turn away transferring his attentions elsewhere, and return later that day or the next.

In the natural system a stallion will cover a mare up to 8–10 times in 24 hours. Nature's system works extremely well resulting in high pregnancy rates per oestrus period. It is a system, however, which is rarely practised today, and is only occasionally seen in pony studs, or with horses run on large expanses of land with minimum involvement from man. One of the problems is that for such a system to run completely naturally the stallion will only cover the mares within his harem and no outside mares can be introduced solely for covering. This can cause difficulties as most studs require visiting mares to be covered by their stallions in order to increase the stud income. The introduction of outside mares in this type of 'natural' system can result in jealousy and hostility from mares within the system, and uncertainty between the stallion and the outside mares. Hence most studs control the covering of their own and visiting mares, often in an intensive, 'in-hand' mating system.

4.2.2 Mating in-hand

Close management of mating is practised on the vast majority of studs today, and is normally termed in-hand mating and involves the complete control of the events of covering. In this and in many other ways, we now control the life of the horse to such an extent that there is little similarity between their natural state and the way most horses now live.

Many studs separate their fillies and colts early on in their lives, sometimes from birth and often at weaning. In the 'natural' system colts and fillies run out together and interact with each other as part of a herd. Youngsters are disciplined by other members of the group and they learn respect at a young age when the chance of serious injury is reduced. One of the problems of intensive systems is that social interaction of young stallions with fillies and mares is removed. In-hand mating then expects stallions to cover mares that they do not know in the highly charged atmosphere of covering, it is not surprising therefore, that the risks of the mare rejecting the stallion and of injury to both parties are high. Many stallions are very valuable, worth tens or hundreds of thousands of pounds. All these issues lead to a very controlled covering process. In addition to this comes the problem of determining when a mare is in oestrus. In the natural system the stallion detects mares in oestrus by using smell and taste but humans have to rely on sight, that is, on observing the behaviour of the mare. This can prove inaccurate, hence most studs use a teaser stallion.

4.2.2.1 Teasing

The teaser stallion is an entire stallion, often of low value, possibly a pony, used under controlled conditions to detect whether a mare is in oestrous or not, but he is not allowed to cover her. Once the teaser stallion has confirmed that the mare is in oestrus she can then be prepared and covered by the stallion of your choice. This means that the stallion used to cover the mares only goes near mares that are confirmed to be in oestrus and so greatly reduces the risk that he will be damaged by a dioestrus mare. Occasionally, less valuable stallions are used to tease the mares they will cover but, the close management of teasing means that they are still protected from damage.

There are problems associated with in-hand covering, the main one being that in their natural state courtship between the stallion and the mare is long but teasing is concentrated into a short period of time and forces the attentions of the stallion upon the mare. Some mares object to this even if they are in oestrus, and so it can be difficult to determine whether they are in oestrus or not. Problems are often encountered with mares with foals at foot. Such mares often object, occasionally violently, to the removal of the foal before teasing and covering, a practice normally done to protect the foal. In the natural system the foal stays close to the mare, but appears to know instinctively to keep its distance. Teasing some mares before feeding or turnout or if it is very hot, cold, raining, windy etc. can be inaccurate, as these conditions may upset the mares and make them reluctant to show oestrus. Some mares need a longer time to be teased, this can be a problem in a busy stud working to a tight schedule and they may never seem to be ready to cover. Again, some mares will only show oestrus under certain conditions, i.e. in the covering yard, when being washed ready for covering, tail bandaged, or when a twitch is applied. It is a good idea, therefore, to have detailed mare records and if you are aware that your mare shows some of these characteristics to let the stud owner/groom know before you have her covered.

There are a wide range of methods used to tease mares, depending on the stud, the value of the stock and the facilities available. In all of the methods the typical signs of oestrus, docility and acceptance of the stallion are looked for.

One of the most common methods of teasing is the use of a trying or teasing board. The mare and stallion are introduced one on either side of the board and their reactions monitored (Figure 4.1(a)–(d)). The

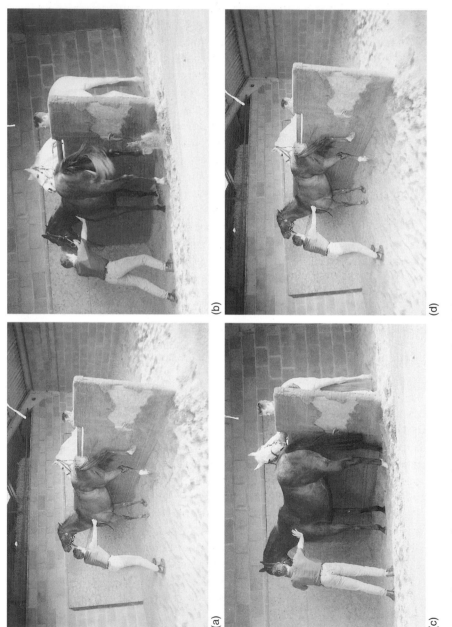

(a)

(b)

(c)

(d)

Figure 4.1 (a)–(d) A mare being teased over a trying or teasing board. The mare and stallion should be introduced initially muzzle to muzzle and the stallion allowed to work his way down the body to the mare's vulva (a), (b), (c). If she is in oestrus she will show little, if any objection. A mare not in oestrus will usually object violently (d). (Photograph Elizabeth Wood, © CABI.)

board is designed to provide protection for both and should be high enough to allow just the horses' heads and necks to reach over. It must be solid in construction, often made of wood, and ideally twice the length of the horses. Its top should be covered by curved rubber or equivalent, to provide protection if the stallion or mare attempt to attack each other over the board. The approach of the teaser to the mare over the board should mimic that of the natural approach. Initially muzzle to muzzle, the teaser is then allowed to stretch his muzzle along the mare's neck, possibly gently nipping her. The attitude of the mare to this attention is closely observed, signs of hostility including laid back ears, squealing, biting and kicking out, indicate that the mare is still in dioestrus (Figure 4.1(d)). In contrast, leaning towards the stallion, rising the tail and the other typical signs of oestrus, indicate that she is ready to be covered (Figure 4.1(a) and (b)). If the mare is interested, then her flank can be turned towards the trying board and the teaser allowed to work his way further down her body (Figure 4.1(c)). It is, however, very important that direct contact with the mare's genital area is avoided to prevent disease transfer to the stallion and then on to other mares to be teased. After a few minutes of such attention most mares will show definite signs of whether or not they are in oestrus, although some mares may require longer.

Using the same principle, a stable door may be used as an alternative, with the teaser in the stable and the mare introduced to him outside. This is a popular practice in the smaller native-type studs, but can be dangerous unless the temperament of the teaser is well known and he is unlikely to get too excited (Figure 4.2).

Teasing over the paddock rail provides another alternative. The teaser is led in-hand to the paddock rail of a field containing mares, which are running loose, normally in small groups. A permanent 'trying' board can be built into the paddock rail or a movable 'trying' board placed there. The reaction of the mares to the teaser is noted. Most mares in oestrus will approach the teaser and show definite signs of oestrus, others may show hostility, some may appear disinterested. Mares which show no reaction, often due to shyness or low social ranking, can be caught and brought up to the trying board and tested individually. Those which show interest can also be teased individually to confirm they are ready for immediate covering. This is an efficient method for use with mares which are turned out as it greatly reduces time and labour and so is popular on bigger studs. A version of this is to just walk (in-hand or ridden) the teaser past the mare paddocks as part of his daily exercise routine. Mares which show interest can then be caught and taken to the covering yard. The system is not so popular with mares and foals due to the perceived risk to foals. Normally however the foals distance themselves from any teasing

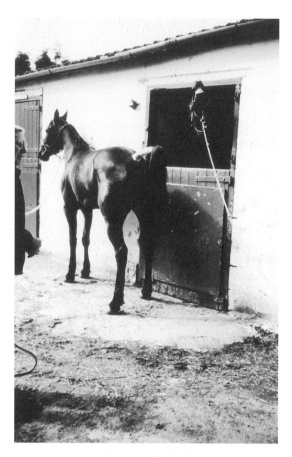

Figure 4.2 Providing it is known that a stallion is good tempered, he may tease mares he is to cover over his stable door. © CABI.

activity (as they do in the natural system) and mares, especially in small groups, are very careful to avoid damage to their foals.

In the southern hemisphere, in places such as South Africa, South America and parts of Australia, mares tend to run in large herds, and are handled less frequently. In such systems mares may be run into chutes or crates and held individually for a short period of time and teased by a stallion standing outside. This system reduces labour and enables large numbers of mares to be teased over a short a period of time, however, the mares must be familiar with this system or errors can occur (Figure 4.3).

Finally, a teasing pen may be used, particularly for shy mares or those which are difficult to tease using other methods. In this system the teaser is confined in a stable or railed area in the corner of a paddock or yard (Figure 4.4). The boards can be tall with a grill or meshed fencing, possibly with a hole through which the teaser can put his head (Figure 4.5). Mares are placed in the paddock or yard and

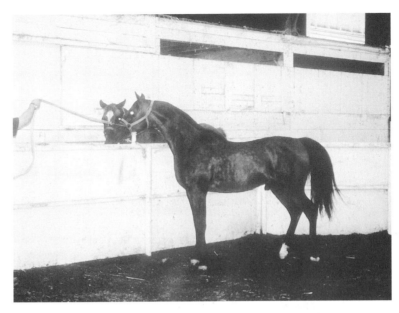

Figure 4.3   Teasing of mares using a chute. Mares may be placed in the crate individually or the crate incorporated as part of a chute system. The stallion is restrained outside the crate and the mares stopped momentarily next to the stallion to gauge their response. (Photograph Julie Baumber, © CABI.)

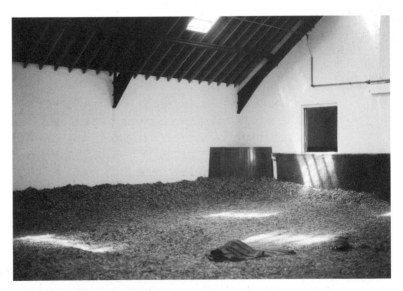

Figure 4.4   An arrangement such as in the photograph above can be used to tease shy or reluctant mares. The stable in the corner of a covering yard (open window in background) is used to confine the teaser, the yard (in the foreground) allows the mare to be free to exhibit oestrus at leisure. (Photograph the National Stud, Newmarket, © CABI.)

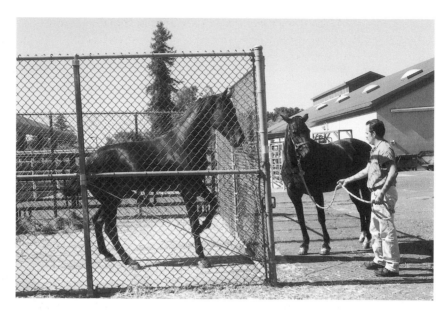

Figure 4.5 A teasing cage, confines the stallion or teaser and allows any mares, either loose within the field or restrained, to approach at will. (Photograph Julie Baumber, © CABI.)

their behaviour towards the teaser noted, as with teasing mares over a paddock rail, those in oestrus will approach the teaser and display signs of oestrus. If a mare is particularly shy she can be placed alone in the paddock or yard and her behaviour monitored. The teaser may also be placed in a central pen with boxes around him in which mares are placed or in a stable adjacent to a mare with a grill between. All these systems work especially well for shy mares, but they are labour intensive as mares need to be watched carefully and these methods do not necessarily avoid direct contact between the genitalia of the mare and the muzzle of the stallion and so all mares must be clear of infection to avoid any disease transfer.

4.2.2.1.1 Teasing mares with a foal at foot

A mare with a foal at foot may present problems at teasing. The foal often becomes agitated at the approach of the stallion and is unaccustomed to the attention he pays to its mother and so distracts her and there is also the fear that valuable foals may be injured. To overcome problems, the foal may either be penned while the mare is being teased, or held within reach or sight of its mother, or removed completely from sight and sound. Knowledge of an individual mare's normal behaviour in such circumstances is very useful as some mares object violently to the removal of the foal.

Not all mares show oestrus under the above systems and some require specific management, prolonged individual teasing etc. The key to success is careful observation, all mares are individuals and no system is completely reliable. Further confirmation of a mare's reproductive state is often required. This is achieved through veterinary examination.

4.2.2.2 Veterinary examination

Veterinary examination, to confirm the stage of the mare's oestrous cycle, is routinely used in many studs, especially when running valuable stallions so that their use can be optimised. Veterinary examination may be used alone, or as a back-up to teasing. There are three types of veterinary examination: ultrasonic scanning, rectal palpation, and vaginal examination. All three techniques are described above (Section 3.2, p. 57). They are used mainly to assess ovarian activity but also the appearance of the uterus, cervix and vagina in order to estimate the likely time of ovulation and therefore establish the best time to cover the mare.

When examining the mare's ovaries the important things to observe are the presence of follicles and/or corpora lutea (CL) along with their size, appearance and position. If an active CL is present then the mare is in dioestrus and it will be some time before she comes into oestrus again. If there are follicles measuring 3.5–4.5 cm in diameter or greater there is a good chance that the mare will ovulate within 48 hours. The size of a follicle is a good guide to the closeness of ovulation, however, some mares ovulate large follicles (6.0–6.5 cm) and some quite small (2.0 cm) ones. A further guide is the feel of the follicle or how it appears at scanning. As a follicle approaches ovulation its wall becomes thinner and it begins to collapse, so at rectal palpation it feels softer and when viewed with a scanner what was previously a clear spherical shape (Figure 3.7, p. 63) now becomes more irregular and the follicle wall appears clearer (Figures 4.6 and 4.7).

Multiple ovulations are an increasing problem in intensively bred mares as modern technology now allows these mares to continue to breed and so pass the trait on to the next generations. The higher the incidence of multiple ovulation the greater the chance of multiple pregnancies and its associated problems (Section 1.4.3.1, p. 29). Scanning mares before covering is an effective way of identifying multiple ovulations and may lead to the decision not to cover that mare. Despite the success of reducing multiple pregnancies to a single one in early pregnancy (Section 5.4, p. 119), some studs still prefer not to cover multiple-ovulating mares and use hormone treatment to bring forward the next oestrus which will hopefully have just the one ovulation.

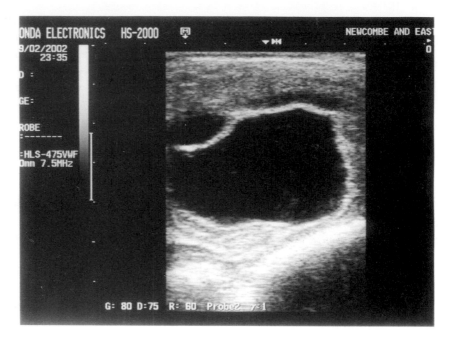

Figure 4.6 An ultrasonic scan of a follicle (4.5 cm wide) immediately before ovulation, notice the thick wall and the loss of a clear, spherical shape. (Photograph Dr John Newcombe, © CABI.)

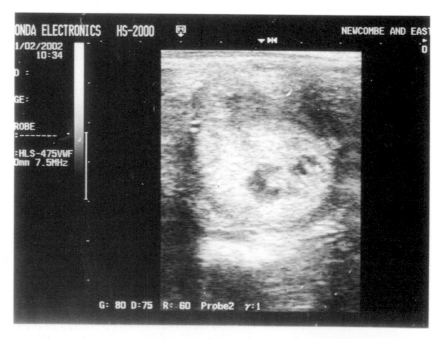

Figure 4.7 An ultrasonic scan of a corpus luteum (CL) immediately after ovulation. (Photograph Dr John Newcombe, © CABI.)

Uterine activity and appearance can also be used as a guide to reproductive activity and is often assessed at the same time as the ovaries at scanning and rectal palpation. Striking changes occur within the uterus between oestrus and dioestrus. As oestrus approaches the uterine endometrial folds become filled with fluid or swollen and can clearly be seen at scanning. The dense central portions of the folds appear white/grey and the swollen portion grey/black giving a characteristic 'sliced orange' or 'cart wheel' appearance, this is a good indicator of approaching ovulation. If rectal palpation is used, the uterine tone and thickness can be felt to increase during dioestrus, the uterus becomes smaller and more flaccid during oestrus.

Finally, examination of the cervix and vagina can give an additional indication of the stage of the cycle but is the least reliable method. By using a vaginascope the cervix during oestrus can be seen to be pink to glistening red in colour, relaxed and 'flowering' into the vagina, which itself also appears red/pink in colour with fluid secretions. During dioestrus the cervix is closed, pale in colour and dry with thick, sticky vaginal secretions, so much so that it is often hard to get the vaginascope into the vagina of a dioestrous mare.

4.2.2.3 Covering

Once it has been determined that the mare is in oestrus and is ready for covering both the mare and the stallion need to be prepared. The exact nature of the preparation will depend upon the system used for mating. Preparation ranges from the strict codes of practice seen in the thoroughbred industry to practically no preparation at all, which is often the case in many native pony studs. The most cautionary preparation will be discussed in the following account though you may find that the stud you choose dispenses with some, if not all, of these preparation techniques. Exact management practice also depends on the size of the stud, labour available etc. In larger studs there are often two to three breeding sessions per day spaced at regular intervals e.g. 9.00 a.m., 2.00 p.m. and 7.00 p.m. Most mares are covered twice within an oestrus, at 24–48 hour intervals or until ovulation has been confirmed.

4.2.2.3.1 The mare
Most big studs will prepare the mare with all eventualities in mind. She is bridled, her tail bandaged and the perineal area thoroughly washed. When washing the mare, gloves should be worn and a new swab of cotton wool should be used for each swipe. Each swipe should be taken from the perineum towards the buttocks and the cotton wool discarded immediately to prevent contamination of the washing solution. If soap is used it should be mild, non-detergent soap and the area

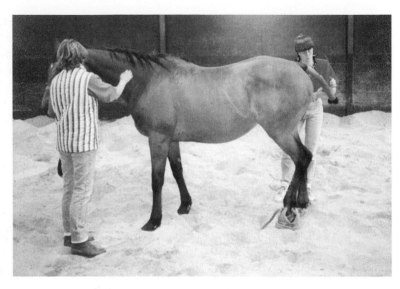

Figure 4.8 A mare ready for covering, tail bandaged, perineum washed and wearing covering boots. (Photograph Angela Stanfield, © CABI.)

should be thoroughly rinsed at the end. Soap and disinfectants kill sperm and may also upset the natural bacterial population of the mare's reproductive tract. At this stage the vulva of mares with a long Caslick should be cut open (episiotomy), covering a mare with a short Caslick is possible with care. Once the mare has been washed she is led to the covering area where felt covering boots may be fitted to her back feet – her hind shoes should have been removed prior to arrival at the stud (Figure 4.8).

The mare may also have a nose or ear twitch applied, depending on her temperament. Some studs twitch as standard, believing that prevention is better than cure as far as damage to expensive stallions is concerned. As a routine on some expensive studs, or if the mare is particularly bad tempered, she may need one of her fore legs held up, or hobbles fitted to prevent her lungeing forward and lashing out when the stallion mounts. Other items, such as blinkers, hood or blindfold, are sometimes used for highly strung maiden or difficult mares. If the mare is to be covered by a stallion with a reputation for biting his mares she can be fitted with a shoulder or whither pad, with or without a biting roll (Figure 4.9).

4.2.2.3.2 The stallion
A stallion's behaviour during the covering season can be unpredictable and, therefore, dangerous. Management techniques can

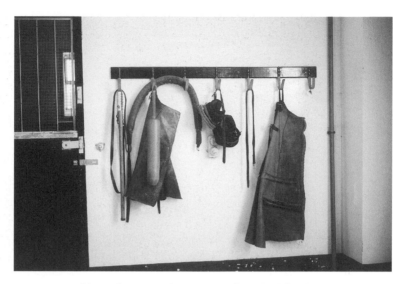

Figure 4.9 Additional items used in covering from the left: a breeding roll, withers pad, covering boots, and neck guard with biting roll. © CABI.

reduce this danger; the most important of these is the use of separate tack for exercise and for covering, so that a stallion is aware of what is required of him by the type of tack used. For covering in intensive, in-hand systems (Section 4.2.2) a stallion is normally tacked up with his covering bridle with a Chiffney or stallion bit and long rein, or a pole may be used to give a greater degree of control.

The stallion is then led from his box to a washing down area where his penis, testes, belly and inside hind legs are washed with warm, clean water (Figure 4.10). Ideally, the penis should be erect at washing. Erection may occur naturally in experienced stallions in anticipation of covering, others may require initial teasing. As with the mare, antiseptic and/or soap solutions, once very popular, should in fact be used with great care due to their detrimental effect on sperm and natural bacterial populations. The stallion is then led to join the mare waiting in the covering area.

4.2.2.3.3 The covering yard

The covering yard can be any area that is quiet, dry and safe with a non-slip surface and away from the mêlée of the general yard. A paddock (Figure 4.11), open yard or covered area specially designed or existing indoor arena may also be used (Figure 4.12).

If an area is to be specially designed it should be at least 20 m by 12 m, roofed, with two sets of wide doors to allow horses to enter and exit in different directions. It is very important that the floor of the cov-

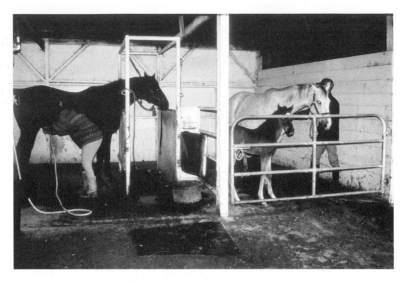

Figure 4.10 Prior to covering, a stallion's penis and genital area should be washed. Erection can be encouraged by the close proximity of an oestrous mare. (Photograph Julie Baumber, © CABI.)

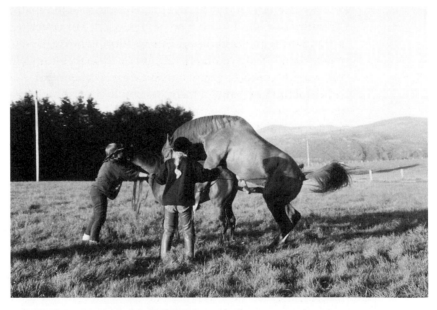

Figure 4.11 Covering in a field or paddock is common practice in smaller studs. (Photograph Gillian Humphries, © CABI.)

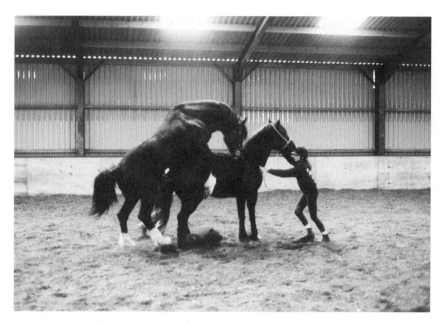

Figure 4.12 The covering yard if large enough can double up as an exercise area. (Photograph Derwen International Welsh Cob Stud, © CABI.)

ering yard is clean, non-slip and dust free. Good surfaces include clay, chalk, peat moss, woodchip, or rubber matting which is currently very popular. The need for a non-slip surface means that floorings such as concrete are not ideal.

4.2.2.3.4 The covering procedure

During covering there should be at least one handler for each horse, wearing stout footwear and a hard hat, the stallion handler should also carry a stick for reprimanding. Traditionally an assistant was present to guide the stallion's penis into the mare if necessary, and/or hold the mare's tail, and a second assistant to hold the stallion steady on the mare. It is essential that all handlers know their exact role and that an emergency procedure has been agreed beforehand. Once she is ready the mare is normally the first to be taken into the covering area. The stallion is then brought in to cover the mare (Figure 4.13 (a)) immediately or in some systems the stallion may initially tease the mare over a trying board within the covering area (Figure 4.13 (b)). This provides him with protection during the initial contact, and is required by some stallions with lower libido in order to avoid a prolonged period with the mare before covering takes place, a potentially dangerous situation.

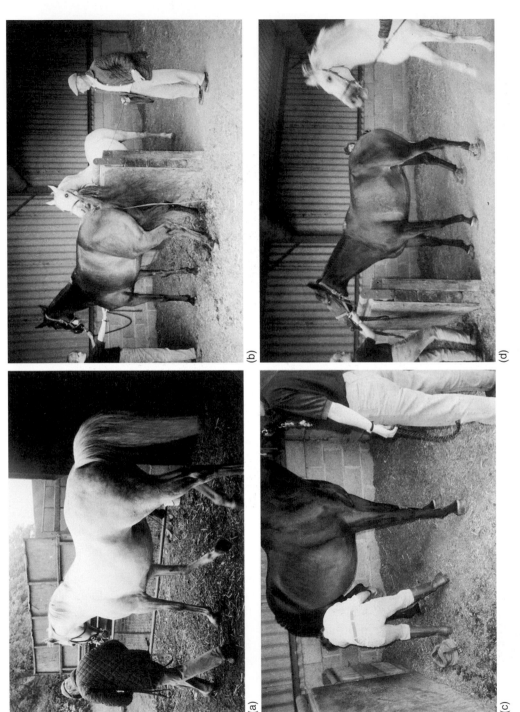

Figure 4.13 (a)–(g) The sequence of events associated with in-hand covering (a) the stallion is bridled and brought into the covering area to meet the mare, (b) the mare may be teased by the stallion over a trying board immediately before covering, (c) covering boots are put on the mare's hind feet, (d) the stallion is allowed to cover the mare, ideally the stallion should be calm and not over enthusiastic, (e) ejaculation is marked by flagging of the stallion's tail, (f) the mare may be stood up against a trying board during covering to prevent her tottering too far forward, (g) ejaculation is followed by a quiescent period prior to dismounting. (Photographs Victoria Kingston, © CABI.)

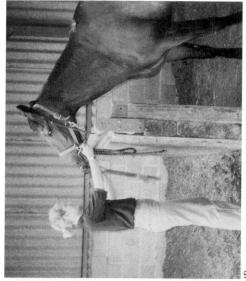

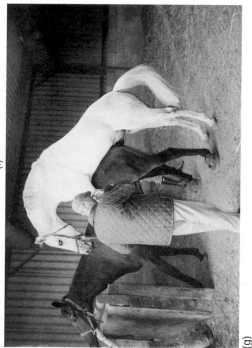

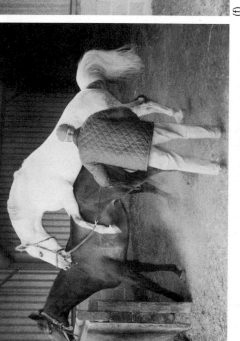

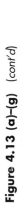

(e)

(f)

(g)

Figure 4.13 (a)–(g) (cont'd)

The mare is then led away from the trying board ready to be covered. At this stage she will have covering boots fitted and may be twitched or hobbled (Figure 4.13 (c)). Once the mare is ready the stallion is allowed to approach her, normally at an angle several feet from her nearside to avoid startling her and causing her to kick out. Once the stallion's penis is fully erect he should be allowed to mount (Figures 4.13 (d) and (e)). Mounting before full erection may damage the stallion.

As the stallion is allowed to mount the mare all handlers should stand on the same side, usually the left. If problems do then occur, both the stallion and the mare can be pulled towards their handlers, turning their hindquarters away from each other and anyone else who is likely to be kicked.

As the stallion mounts the mare she will probably totter forwards. This should be allowed as long as she does not move too far. Excessive tottering can put strain on the stallion, who will rest more of his weight on the mare's back in turn causing her strain or injury. Some studs prevent this by holding the mare up against a protective barrier (Figures 4.13 (d) and (e)). This arrangement may also be used to protect handlers from mares which strike out (Figure 4.13 (f)). If a leg strap is being used to restrain the mare it must be released at this stage.

Many traditional studs still have an assistant stallion handler to pull the mare's tail to one side and guide the penis into the vagina. However, this practice is now frowned upon by many and is seen as excessive interference which may disrupt the normal course of events leading up to ejaculation. Successful ejaculation can normally be seen as rhythmic flagging of the stallion's tail (Figure 4.13 (e)). If in doubt the contractions of the urethra can be felt by placing a hand along the bottom of the penis. After ejaculation, the stallion should be allowed to relax on the mare (Figure 4.13 (g)). During this period of relaxation the glans penis, which has increased in size considerably at ejaculation, returns to normal allowing the penis to be withdrawn. Early withdrawal can damage both the stallion and the mare so he should be allowed to dismount in his own time, which may take several minutes. The mare should then be turned towards her handler and walked slowly away allowing the stallion to slide off and so reducing the chance of him being kicked. The stallion should similarly be turned towards his handler after he has dismounted, again reducing the chance of injury to the mare or handlers. The presence of spermatozoa in dismount semen samples can be used to confirm ejaculation. At this time a 'dismount swab' may also be taken from the urethral area. Increasingly, in studs running high value stallions, the mating process is recorded on a video camera to provide additional evidence that covering has taken place.

After covering the stallion should be allowed to relax and then walked to the washing area, where his penis should be washed and his genitalia examined for abrasions. Many studs walk mares around slowly after covering in the belief that this prevents straining which causes the loss of valuable semen. However, as the vast majority of the semen is deposited into the top of the cervix and into the uterus a significant loss of semen is very unlikely.

Occasionally the mare and stallion differ in size; this can be accommodated by having a dip in the floor or by using a breeding platform to equal the horse's heights. In the US hydraulic breeding platforms are used which can be adjusted to the exact height required. Mating horses which vary greatly in size should be done with care. A very large stallion put on to a small mare may cause her problems in late pregnancy due to the large size of the fetus.

4.2.2.3.5 Management of covering during foal heat

Teasing and covering mares with foals at foot can be challenging (Section 4.2.2.1.1, p. 86). The majority of mares either foal at stud or arrive at the stud with foals of a very young age. In nature, the presence of a foal presents no problems as foals naturally move away from mating activity but stay within sight of the mare. As with teasing, if mating is to occur in a large open area, the foal may be let loose and will normally keep well away from the proceedings, but within sight of its dam, reducing anxiety and stress. If mating is to occur in a small, enclosed covering yard, or if the mare is difficult, the foal should be restrained for its own safety. It may be best to put it in a box or cage within sight of the mare and with a handler to watch it. However, some mares will become distracted by the antics of the foal. In such cases it may be better to remove the foal completely, out of sight and earshot. The system used depends entirely on the character of the mare and foal, the facilities available and personal preference.

4.2.3 Alternative natural covering methods

As mentioned previously, there are many variations in covering practice. Many methods are cost effective and used on the smaller native studs where nomination fees are cheaper, for example native ponies successfully cover mares in-hand in a convenient field near to the main yard. This is how mares would have been covered in the past, when stallions were walked from farm to farm. If covering is to occur in a large field then the stallion used must be well behaved and controlled, as his escape may cause serious problems with neighbouring mares.

Pasture breeding is another alternative, popular in South Africa and South America and also Iceland, where mares are run in large herds over wide expanses of land. In such systems stallions are turned out to run free with a group of mares and to cover them at will. This system is the nearest to the natural situation but, as discussed (Section 4.2.1, p. 79) presents problems with visiting mares. A 'half-way house' between in-hand breeding and pasture breeding is to allow the stallion to be loose in the field and introduce mares to him individually, either restrained or free. This system allows the stallion to be used efficiently but allows visiting mares to be covered in a near natural system. Stallions used in this system must be well behaved and, especially if the mare is restrained, their characteristics should be well known to the mare handler, so that any necessary avoiding action may be taken. Turning a stallion out with an individual mare is a popular method in native pony studs and can be used to get problem mares in foal.

4.3 ARTIFICIAL INSEMINATION

There are many reasons why you may choose to use AI to cover your mare. The most common is that it will allow you to use a stallion which is some distance away, or even abroad, and so increase the range of stallions available and reduce the risks and expense of travel. However, AI may also be chosen to:

- minimise disease transfer by using antibiotic extenders;
- increase the chance of conception in mares susceptible to uterine endometritis;
- reduce the risk of injury to humans and stock especially if the mare or stallion is particularly nervous;
- breed difficult mares and stallions, i.e. those with physical abnormalities especially those caused by accidents, infection, poor perineal conformation, psychological problems, etc. However, care must always be taken to ensure that such problems are not hereditary.
- from the stallion owner's point of view AI increases the number of mares he can cover per season and hence improves financial return.

Much of the paperwork involved, especially certificates to confirm disease-free status etc., are the same in AI as they are for in-hand covering (Sections 3.4.1, p. 69, 3.4.2, p. 71, 3.5.1, p. 76). However, additional paperwork will be required, particularly if semen is being imported/exported. It is, therefore, essential that before embarking on AI you contact the relevant Breed Society to ascertain their regulations and obtain the necessary paperwork. They should also be able to provide you with a list of stallions available by AI. Using this information a stallion can be chosen and the Breed Society's requirements discussed with the veterinary surgeon and/or inseminator in good time. It should be noted, however, that although the vast majority of breed societies do accept the use of AI there is one major exception, the Thoroughbred Breed Society, which does not register any stock conceived by AI.

AI is based upon the principle of collecting semen from a stallion, extending it with a specifically formulated extender (Section 4.3.2, p. 203), which allows for varying lengths of storage time and/or transport, followed by insemination into the mare.

4.3.1 Semen collection

The most common method of semen collection is via an artificial vagina (AV) (Figures 4.14 and 4.15 (a) and (e)). The AV mimics the mare's vagina. It consists of a warm sterile tube (known as a lumen) surrounded by a water jacket, under some pressure, plus a collecting vessel. The water jacket is filled with warm water to ensure a lumen temperature of 44–48°C. The pressure within the AV can be adjusted by increasing or decreasing the volume of water or by pumping in air. The collecting vessel should also be warm (38–44°C) to prevent cold shock which is fatal to sperm.

An oestrus mare or dummy is used to encourage the stallion to ejaculate into the AV (Figure 4.15 (a)–(k)). If a mare is to be used, covering occurs as for natural service except that the stallion's penis is diverted into the AV rather than entering the mare's vagina (Figure 4.15 (f)). A dummy provides a safer alternative and most stallions can be trained to use one (Figure 4.15 (k)).

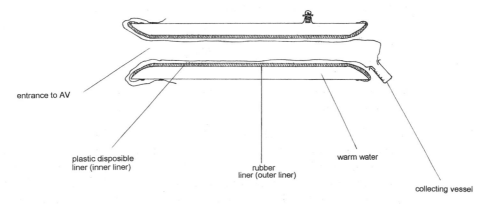

entrance to AV

plastic disposible liner (inner liner)

rubber liner (outer liner)

warm water

collecting vessel

Figure 4.14 A diagram of an artificial vagina (AV).

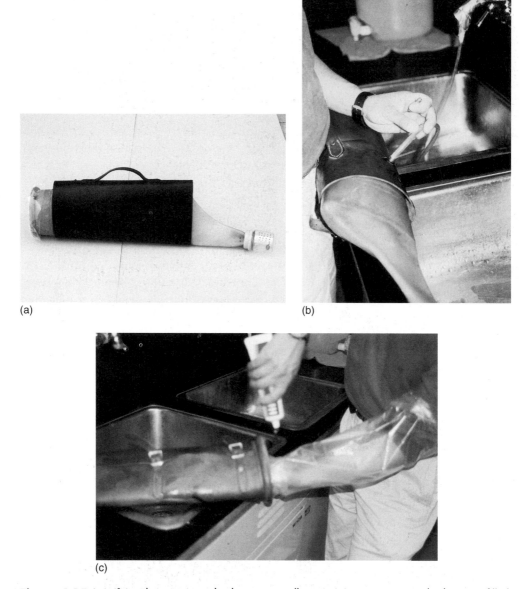

(a)

(b)

(c)

Figure 4.15 (a)–(k)   The events involved in semen collection: (a) a Missouri AV; (b) the AV is filled with warm water to ensure a lumen temperature of 44–48°C; (c) lubrication of the AV; (d) introduction or teasing of the stallion and mare; (e) AV ready for use; (f) guiding the stallion's penis into the AV. Note the correct positioning of handlers all on the same side of the mare and stallion; (g) slightly inclined positioning of the AV to mimic the natural angle of the mare's vagina; (h) dismount of the stallion and slow removal of the AV ensuring all semen is collected; (i) after dismount the stallion should be turned away from the mare to reduce the risk of injury; (j) the collected sample; (k) semen collection using dummy. (Photographs Julie Baumber and Victor Medinal, © CABI.)

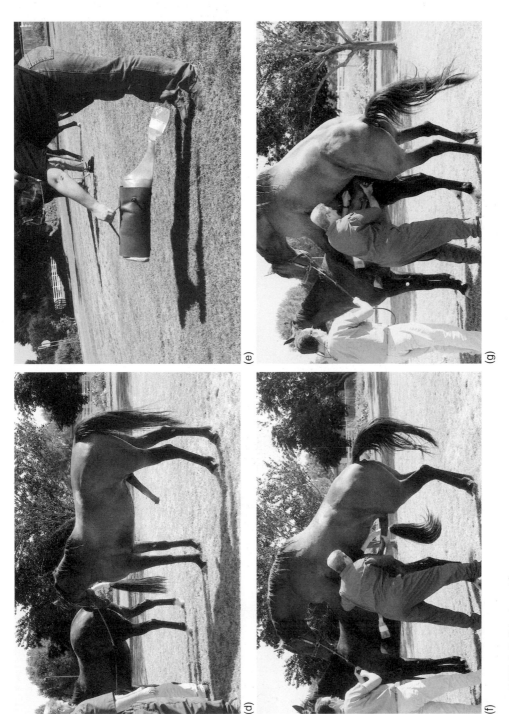

(d)

(e)

(f)

(g)

Figure 4.15 (a)–(k) (cont'd)

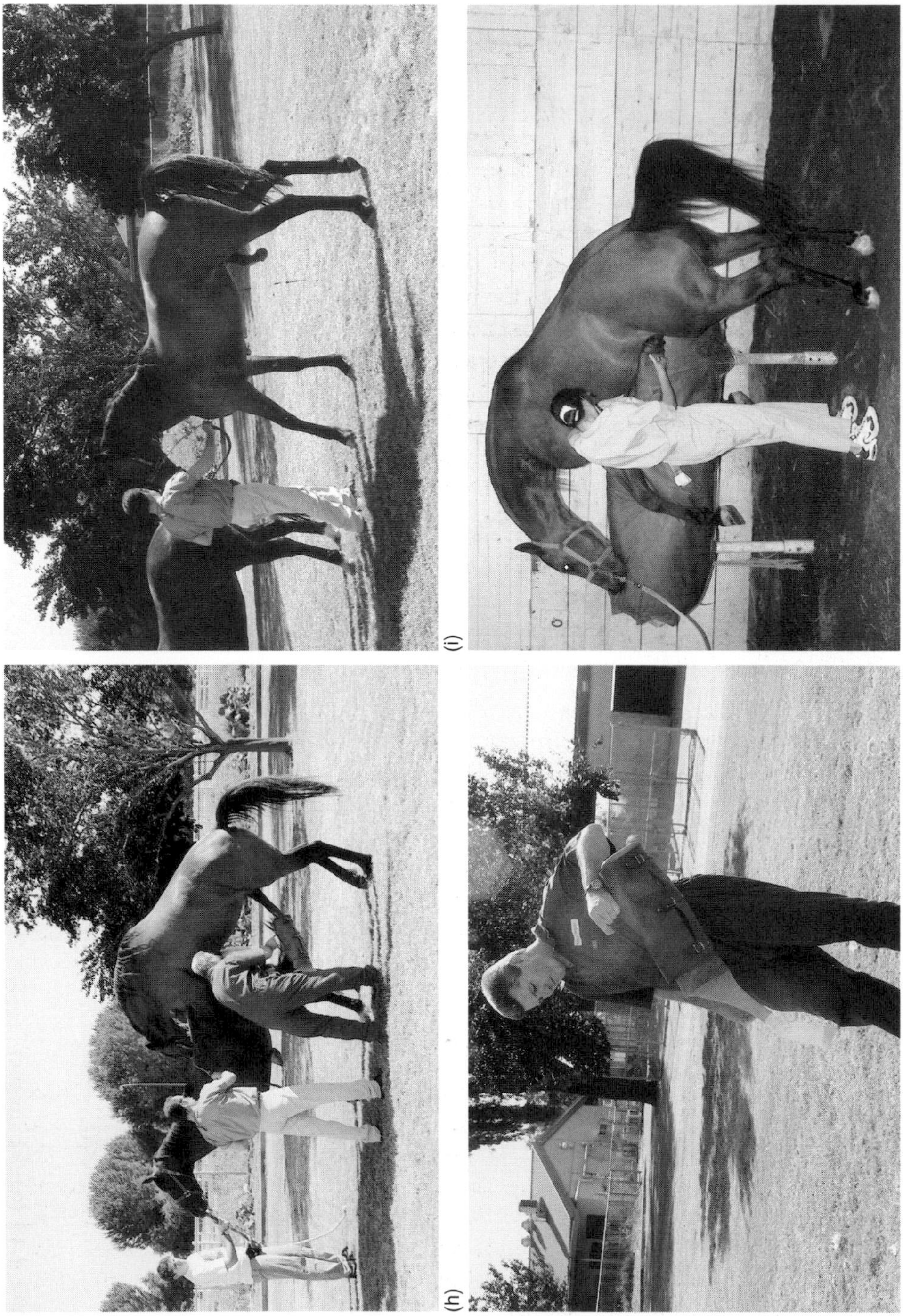

Figure 4.15 (a)–(k) *(cont'd)*

Once the semen has been collected it must be kept at body temperature (38°C) until it has been evaluated and either used immediately or extended (see below) and stored.

4.3.2 Semen evaluation

Immediately after collection and before storage the semen must be evaluated to determine its quality. Sperm concentration and progressive motility (the percentage of sperm moving in a forward direction) are nearly always assessed to give an indication of the number of live sperm present and hence the number of insemination doses which can be obtained. Morphology (number of normal sperm), percentage of live sperm, cytology (presence of white and red blood cells), pH, longevity (i.e. how long the sperm survive in an incubator) and bacteriology may also be assessed, especially if the semen is destined for export, or at the beginning of each season, or if a problem is suspected. The semen sample arriving for use with a mare should have been assessed at collection and an evaluation report should be included with the sample along with disease certification, giving a quality guarantee.

4.3.3 Semen extension and storage

There are three types of semen which might be available for your mare, fresh, chilled or frozen. Before semen is stored for any length of time it needs to have an *extender* added to provide extra nutrients to support the sperm, in particular more energy, and so prolong the sperms' life. In the absence of an extender the nutrients of the seminal plasma, which naturally provide the sperm with support, are soon used up. A variety of extenders can be used, though most are based upon non-fat dried skimmed milk solids, skimmed milk, or occasionally egg yolk.

4.3.3.1 Fresh semen

Fresh, or raw, semen remains in the state it was when collected from the stallion and normally with no extender and so will not survive more than a few hours. It must be kept at body temperature (38°C) and used immediately; in this case, the stallion and mare need to be on the same yard. This method is not popular because of the limited lifespan of the semen sample but it is sometimes used with problem or difficult mares, or if a stallion is due to cover too many mares in one day for natural service.

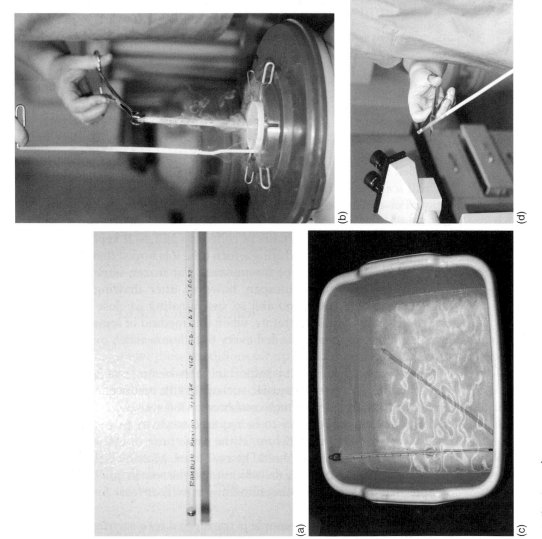

Figure 4.17 (a)–(i) (cont'd)

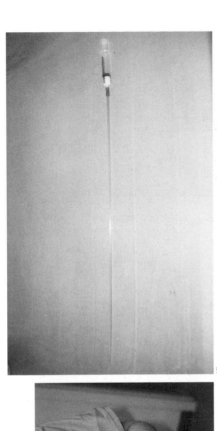

(f)

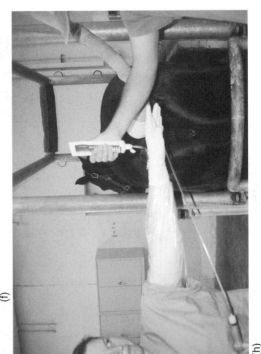

(h)

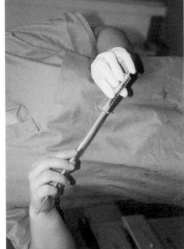

(e)

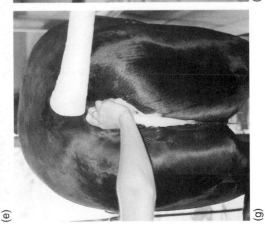

(g)

Figure 4.17 (a)–(i) *(cont'd)*

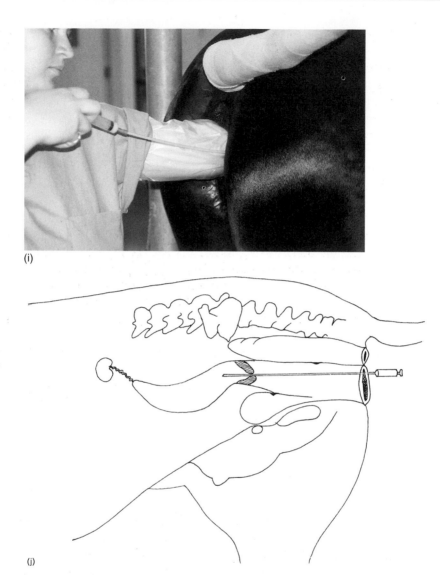

(i)

(j)

Figure 4.17 (a)–(j) *(cont'd)* Techniques used to inseminate a mare: (a) a plastic round straw is one of the most common methods of storing frozen semen; (b) frozen semen is stored in liquid nitrogen flasks, from which it must be removed for thawing immediately before insemination; (c) a large straw of frozen semen thawing in warm water immediately before insemination; (d) after thawing, the ends of the straw are cut; (e) semen from either a single straw or a number of straws is then drained into the syringe; (f) the syringe is attached to the end of the insemination pipette in readiness for insemination; (g) prior to insemination the mare should be prepared, perineal area washed, tail bandaged and then held in stocks; (h) a small amount of lubricant should be placed on the hand; (i) the hand should be introduced slowly into the vagina along with the insemination pipette, when the pipette is in place, the plunger of the syringe is slowly depressed to expel all the semen into the uterus; (j) diagram illustrating the correct position of the insemination pipette for depositing the semen. (Embryos may be transferred non-surgically into donor mares in a similar manner.) (Photographs Julie Baumber and Victor Medina, © CABI.)

for chilled semen. For smaller volume straws (0.5–1 ml) (Figure 4.17 (a)) specially designed insemination guns allow the straw to be held within the gun and the semen expelled directly when the plunger is pushed. Whatever the volume of frozen semen used, approximately 800 million sperm will be inseminated at a time, more than for chilled semen, to compensate for any loss occurring during the freezing process.

The act of insemination is relatively simple, and regardless of whether the semen is frozen, chilled or fresh the technique is the same (Figure 4.17 (c)–(j)). The mare should be restrained in stocks with her perineal area washed and tail bandaged (Figure 4.17 (g)). The inseminator will insert an insemination pipette or gun, with the aid of their lubricated hand and forearm, into the vagina, up through the cervix and into the uterus using their forefinger (Figure 4.17 (i) and (j)). As an alternative the inseminator may guide the insemination pipette through the cervix by feeling through the rectum wall, as in rectal palpation. This method is preferred by some as it is thought to run a lower risk of infection since only the fine insemination pipette enters the mare's reproductive tract.

Once the pipette is in place within the uterus the syringe plunger is slowly pushed to expel the sample.

AI is a relatively easy, safe and convenient method of covering mares with stallions from all over the world. As with all techniques it has its positive and negative points, however, used sensibly, its future as a technique for breeding horses is assured.

4.4 CONCLUSION

There are a number of management practices for covering mares both by natural mating or AI. The system used is decided by the mare owner, the individual stud, its facilities, normal practices and labour available. Financial considerations also dictate management choices. Intensive in-hand breeding systems are increasingly popular, providing maximum protection for both handlers and horses, but often at the expense of natural behaviour and reproductive performance. AI has yet to take off as a major means of covering mares within the UK despite its popularity elsewhere in the world, largely due to the refusal of the Thoroughbred Breeders' Association to register any progeny conceived by AI.

Management of the Pregnant Mare

5

5.1 INTRODUCTION

Management of the pregnant mare is particularly important during the initial and latter stages of pregnancy, in order to ensure the well-being of the mare and the foal. The vast majority of pregnancies develop within the mare in which they were conceived, however, occasionally embryo transfer is used in which case one mare conceives the pregnancy but the embryo develops in the uterus of another.

5.2 EMBRYO TRANSFER

The main principle behind embryo transfer (ET) is the transfer of an embryo from a valuable donor mare mated to a valuable stallion into an ordinary mare, but one which will provide the foal with the best uterine environment and the best start in life. The genetic make-up of the mare carrying the foal has no effect on the characteristics of that foal, which will continue to carry the genetic make-up of its genetic mother and father. The first equine ET was carried out in Japan in 1974, however, its use is still not widespread largely due to cost, it can cost several thousand pounds per foal. However, in some circumstances, such as for polo ponies in Argentina, it is more widely used. One of the major problems, apart from the cost, is the continued reluctance of breed societies to register ET foals.

5.2.1 Reasons for using ET

There are many reasons why you may choose to use ET with your mare, these include:

- to obtain foals from mares which are unable to carry a foal or go through the strain of foaling;
- to obtain foals from older mares without risk;
- to provide a genetically promising foal with the best uterus and start in life (including mothering ability and milk production in the recipient mare);
- to allow performance mares to breed without interrupting their career;
- to freeze embryos for future use or for export/import;
- to aid in the breeding of exotic equids;
- to increase the number of foals/mare/lifetime;
- to allow cloning, embryo sexing etc.

5.2.2 Donor and recipient mares

In order for embryo transfer to be successful, the uterus into which the embryo is transferred must be at the same stage in the reproductive cycle as the uterus from which it was collected. To achieve this, the oestrous cycles of the donor and recipient mares must be synchronised, this is normally achieved through hormone therapy (Section 2.2.1.2.2, p. 45). Ideally, recipient mares are five to ten years old with a proven breeding record and no history of uterine infection or any other reproductive problems, they should be larger than the donor, to give the fetus the largest possible uterus and so allow maximum growth before birth. Large mares such as draft animals are popular as recipients not only due to their size but also because of their placid easy temperament. Some companies will rent out recipient mares for a fee.

5.2.3 Embryo recovery

Once ovulation in the donor mare has been confirmed, usually by scanning, she is covered naturally or by AI. The method of embryo collection depends on the age of the embryos to be recovered. In commercial practice equine embryos are normally collected by non-surgical collection at eight days (Figure 5.1).

5.2.3.1 Non-surgical recovery

Non-surgical recovery is the usual commercial method for collecting embryos of six to eight days of age as it is non-invasive and there is no need for a general anaesthetic and it therefore carries lower risks. The mare is restrained in stocks, with the perineal area washed and tail bandaged. A catheter is inserted through the mare's cervix and into the uterus (Figure 5.1).

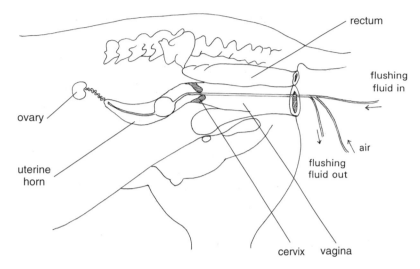

Figure 5.1 Embryo transfer in the mare, illustrating the catheter in place ready for flushing and collection of embryos. © CABI.

The catheter is passed as high as possible up into each uterine horn in turn. Once in position, the cuff of the catheter is inflated via the inlet tube which blocks the base of the uterine horn, preventing the escape of the flushing medium through the uterus (Figure 5.1). Fluid is then flushed in through the entry catheter into the top of the uterine horn, and returns, along with any embryos present, through the outlet tube, where it is collected in a warm collecting vessel (Figure 5.1).

5.2.3.2 Surgical recovery

Surgical recovery is a less popular method of embryo transfer as it is invasive and is carried out under general anaesthetic or sedation, but it does allow younger (up to Day 5) and more robust embryos to be collected which give better pregnancy rates. The mare is anaesthetised and laid on her back (dorsal recumbency) (Figure 5.2). The uterus is accessed through a hole made in the abdomen wall and a ligature tied around the top of the uterine horn to prevent fluid escaping. A glass tube is then inserted into the end of the horn just above the ligature. Fluid is flushed, through a blunt-ended needle inserted into the top of the fallopian tube, down towards the uterine horn. As the fluid passes, it washes out any embryos and exits through the glass tube at the end of the uterine horn and into a warm collecting vessel.

Both methods of recovery have their advantages and disadvantages. Surgical recovery allows younger, more robust embryos to be col-

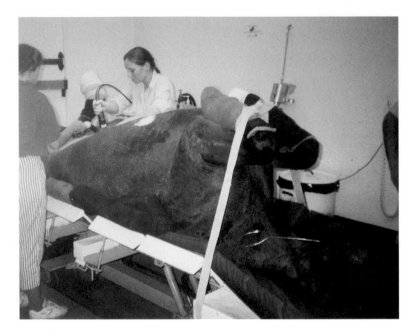

Figure 5.2 A mare prepared for surgical embryo recovery.

lected, but at a greater risk to the mare. Non-surgical recovery allows older (Day 6 onwards), less robust embryos to be collected, but with a lower risk to the mare and with potential for multiple recoveries.

5.2.4 Embryo evaluation

Once collected, the embryo must be evaluated to ensure that it is in fact fertilised and at the correct stage of development for its age. Embryos are graded on a scale from one to five, one being excellent and five dead, grade three or better are suitable for transfer. Throughout the evaluation process it is essential that embryos are kept warm (35–38°C) and that all equipment used is also pre-warmed and sterile.

5.2.5 Embryo storage

Normally, recovered embryos are transferred immediately, or chilled for transportation. If they are to be used within the next few hours they can be kept at body temperature, for transportation they can be cooled and kept at 4–5°C for 36–48 hours. In the commercial sector embryos can be cooled, stored and transported in an Equitainer (Figure 4.16, p. 104) which acts like a cool box. The only possibility for long-term storage is freezing; however this has not been very successful in horses, the first foal from a frozen embryo was born in 1982. There is some suggestion that younger embryos freeze better, hence surgical collection is often used if embryos are to be frozen.

5.2.6 Embryo transfer

The transfer of embryos can, as with collection, be done either surgically or non-surgically.

5.2.6.1 Non-surgical embryo transfer

The non-surgical transfer of embryos is very similar to the techniques used in AI (Section 4.3.4, p. 105). The mare is restrained within stocks, the perineal area thoroughly washed, the transfer gun or catheter with attached syringe, containing the embryo is passed through the mare's cervix and into the uterine body (Figure 4.17 (j)). Once in place, the embryo and fluids are expelled into the uterus by slowly pushing the plunger of the syringe.

Non-surgical transfer is a relatively easy and quick procedure. However, it can only be used for embryos of six days and older (those which would have naturally passed into the uterus from the fallopian tube) and it does run an increased risk of introducing infections into the reproductive tract.

5.2.6.2 Surgical embryo transfer

Surgical transfer is not as widespread today but is sometimes used with frozen embryos, allowing embryos younger than five days of age to be placed at the very top of the uterine horn. As with surgical embryo collection, a general anaesthetic or sedation is required. The mare is prepared in a similar way as for surgical collection but a smaller incision is made. Only the uterine horn is accessed through the incision and a small hole is made at the top of the horn with a blunt needle. A pipette, containing the embryo, is pushed through this hole into the top of the uterine horn and the embryo expelled from the pipette.

5.3 PREGNANCY DETECTION

Regardless of the means of conception, natural or ET, the mare needs to be confirmed as pregnant as soon as possible so that she can be managed correctly or if necessary re-covered. Early detection also allows twin pregnancies to be diagnosed and appropriate action taken

(Section 5.4, p. 119). It may also be necessary for sale or for insurance purposes or if the nomination agreement is 'no foal no fee October 1' (Section 3.4.2, p. 71).

The mnemonic A.E.I.O.U. describes the major requirements of an ideal pregnancy test:

A – Accurate
E – Early
I – Inexpensive
O – Once only
U – Uncomplicated

Unfortunately, although there are numerous methods of detecting pregnancy, none as yet meet all these criteria.

5.3.1 Manual methods of pregnancy detection

Manual methods of pregnancy detection are the oldest and cheapest and still in common use. Their major advantage is that they give an immediate result, though they can only be accurately used after Day 20 of pregnancy. Examination is via rectal palpation or cervical/vaginal examination. Rectal palpation (Section 3.2, p. 57) allows the uterus to be felt through the rectum wall and, with experience, accurate diagnosis can be made at Day 20–30 when the swelling of the uterus around the conceptus can first be felt. The most accurate results are from Day 60, at which stage the age of the fetus can be estimated to within one week and the presence of twins detected. In late pregnancy it becomes possible to feel fetal structures, such as the head and ribs through the uterine wall. Table 5.1 indicates the size of the conceptus at various stages in early pregnancy.

Table 5.1   The size of the embryonic vesicle at stages during early pregnancy in the mare.

Age of pregnancy (days post conception)	Average embryonic vesicle size (diameter mm)	Comments
12	9–11	Earliest detection by ultrasound
14	12–16	
15	16–20	
20	30–40	Embryo first detected and heartbeat seen on ultrasound
30	40–50	
40	65	
50	80	
60	100–130	Most accurate diagnosis via rectal palpation

The major disadvantage of rectal palpation is that it cannot be accurately used early enough to detect mares which have failed to conceive in time to allow them to be re-covered at the next oestrus. However, the technique is quick, simple, cheap and gives immediate results.

Vaginascopy allows the mare's cervix to be examined (Section 3.2, p. 57) and may be used as an aid to pregnancy detection, however, it is not accurate enough to be used alone and so is used to support rectal palpation. In the pregnant mare the cervix should appear white/light pink in colour, and should be firm with sticky mucous.

5.3.2 Blood tests

Blood tests are used in small ponies and mares with an injury or rectal/vaginal tears, where rectal palpation and ultrasonic detection are not advisable. Blood plasma concentrations of one or several hormones (equine chorionic gonadotropin (eCG), progesterone and oestrogen) are measured. These tests can be very accurate but are expensive and there is a delay before the results are available. ECG (also known as pregnant mare serum gonadotropin, PMSG) is secreted by the endometrial cups between Days 40 and 100 of pregnancy (Section 2.2.2.1, p. 48). The test for eCG is accurate but is unable to determine whether or not the fetus is alive, as the endometrial cups continue to secrete eCG for a short time after fetal death. Progesterone is known as the hormone of pregnancy, high concentrations are required if pregnancy is to be maintained (Section 2.2.2.1, p. 48) and therefore its presence indicates that the mare is pregnant. Progesterone can be tested for as early as Day 16–17, when levels higher than 3–4 ng/ml suggest that the mare is pregnant. In non-pregnant mares progesterone levels at this time should be dropping. However, oestrous cycle abnormalities such as prolonged dioestrus can result in high progesterone levels for longer and so be mistaken for pregnancy. Kits for the rapid testing of plasma progesterone concentrations are available commercially. Finally, oestrogen levels can be measured. High levels from Day 85–210 indicate that the mare is pregnant.

Blood tests can be useful but are limited to use relatively late in pregnancy or in the case of progesterone have limited accuracy.

5.3.3 Milk tests

Although blood hormone concentrations are most commonly used, there may be occasions in lactating mares when obtaining a milk sample is easier and less stressful for the mare. Both progesterone and oestrogen can be detected in the milk of a pregnant mare and follow the same pattern as in blood. Progesterone is the major hormone used for pregnancy testing, with commercial kits available; however, there is the same problem as with blood sampling in differentiating between pregnancy and abnormal cycles in early pregnant mares.

5.3.4 Urine and faeces tests

Urine and faeces tests are not widely used but do have their uses in non-lactating mares where rectal palpation or blood sampling proves difficult or in wild animals. Samples are tested for oestrogen which, as with blood samples, is detected from about Day 90 (urine) or Day 120 (faeces) to Day 200.

5.3.5 Ultrasonic pregnancy detection

Since the 1980s ultrasonic scanning has revolutionised the detection of pregnancy in many animals particularly the mare. Ultrasonic detection (Section 3.2, p. 57) gives an immediate result and can be carried out on the stud as the equipment is fully portable. The uterus is examined and the conceptus, if present, can be detected as a discrete spherical sac (Figure 5.3).

The size of the embryonic vesicle at various stages of early pregnancy is given in Table 5.1, p. 116. Pregnancy can first be detected

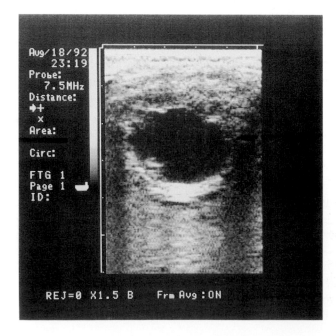

Figure 5.3 A typical scan showing a pregnancy at Day 20. The embryo is evident as a white structure towards the bottom left of the dark fluid-filled area, which is the blastocoel (Section 1.4.2, p. 21). © CABI.

ultrasonically at Day 12, at which stage only the whole conceptus (embryo plus blastocoel and trophoblast) can be identified. At this stage the conceptus moves within the uterus making detection more difficult. By Day 17–18 the conceptus slows down and is normally found at the junction of the uterine body and horn. By Day 20 the embryo itself can be identified within the whole conceptus. At Day 24 the fetal heartbeat can be seen and between Days 59 and 78 the sex of the fetus may be determined.

In practice most studs scan at Day 18, which is the time which gives most accurate results and early enough to allow arrangements to be made for re-covering. A second scan may then be done at Day 40, when the period of highest risk of embryo mortality has passed. Mares are usually sent home after one or other of these scans as long pregnancy is detected, depending on the arrangements at individual studs. In the thoroughbred industry where there is a high incidence of twins, initial scanning is often carried out at Day 12, at which time twins may be identified and if present the mare managed accordingly (Section 5.4, p. 119). The mare is then re-scanned at Days 18–20 and again at Day 40. Scanning can also be used later on in pregnancy to assess fetal viability.

5.4 MANAGEMENT OF TWIN PREGNANCIES

The conception of twins is a significant problem in the management of the pregnant mare as the mare is unable to carry twins to term except on rare occasions (Section 1.4.3.1, Figure 1.30, pp. 29–30). Twinning is the biggest cause of non-infective abortion in mares. It is a real advantage to be able to identify and then manage twin pregnancies as early as possible in the pregnancy. The use of ultrasonic scanning has significantly helped this early identification of twins.

There are four main management practices used to reduce the incidence of twins: monitor ovulation; wait and see; manually reduce; or treat with PGF2α. Historically, rectal palpation was used to detect whether two large follicles were present on the ovary and if so the mare would not be covered on that oestrus. However, many twin pregnancies naturally reduce to singles by Day 20 and so this method was wasting many potential pregnancies. Many studs then allowed covering and monitored any multiple pregnancies to see if natural reduction occurred. If not, abortion was induced at a later stage, but this had the disadvantage that these mares were barren that particular year. The development and use of scanning in the 1980s allowed such monitoring of multiple pregnancies to be done more easily.

An alternative to waiting for natural reduction is to reduce manually; this is the most common practice on studs these days. Manual reduction of twins to a single is reported to be up to 96% successful between Days 13 and 16. It involves the squeezing of the smallest embryo, identified by ultrasound, either between the thumb and forefinger or up against the uterine wall and pelvis using the scanner probe until the vesicle ruptures. This is best done before Day 18 and so is normally carried out at initial scanning on Day 12 if twins are detected. After Day 18 the manual reduction of bilateral twins (one in each horn) can still be very successful but reduction of unilateral twins (both in the same horn) runs a higher risk of losing the whole pregnancy. A final alternative to manual reduction is to induce abortion of the whole pregnancy artificially and start again by re-covering the mare at the next oestrus which can be brought forward using PGF2α.

5.5 MANAGEMENT OF THE PREGNANT MARE

Correct general management of the pregnant mare is important to ensure that the foal is given every advantage and that the mare's future reproductive career is not affected. The mare should be in fit condition throughout pregnancy, this will help ensure that she has an easy foaling and that she will be in good physical condition for her next pregnancy.

5.5.1 Exercise

Exercise and nutrition go hand in hand, and together are the major factors which determine body condition. As with most mares a body condition of 3 is ideal (Section 3.4, p. 66, and Figures 3.9, p. 67 and 3.10, p. 68). The specific amount of exercise depends on the individual mare and her history. A moderate exercise regime can be provided in the form of self exercise by regular turnout in an open field or gentle ridden exercise in early pregnancy (Figure 5.4). Mares which are used to being ridden can be ridden with increasing gentleness up to six months of pregnancy. In the last third of pregnancy forced exercise should stop and be replaced by turn out with a group if possible. Mares turned out in groups tend to exercise more effectively than those turned out alone. Gentle exercise helps: the mare's circulatory system (essential for maintaining blood supply to the placenta); reduces water retention (which causes filled legs, often seen in mares left standing indoors); maintains body condition and reduces obesity (reducing the chances of complications at parturition).

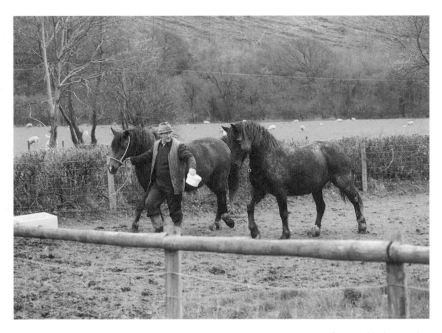

Figure 5.4 Exercise is essential in order to maintain a mare's fitness, body condition score of 3 and to prevent circulatory problems in the later stages of pregnancy. (Photograph Mr Tom James, Penpontbren Stud, © CABI.)

Exercise must always be consistent and not to exhaustion, as this has been associated with stress and abortion.

5.5.2 Nutrition

The nutritional requirements of a pregnant mare vary according to whether she has a foal at foot (lactating), or she was previously barren. The length of lactation in the mare today is determined by man and normally lasts for six to eight months. It is, therefore, during this time that the two groups of mares with or without foals at foot have different requirements. In an ideal system, and providing there are enough mares, these two classes of animals should be kept and fed separately. During pregnancy a mare's body condition and weight should be monitored carefully to ensure that neither excess body condition is gained, nor that she has to use her body reserves to make up for inadequate nutrition. The use of weigh scales is a good way of monitoring weight, however, many people do not have access to one and so a weigh band can be used to indicate weight change (Figure 5.5). A number of equations can also be used but these are less accurate for indicating weight gain or loss especially for pregnant mares.

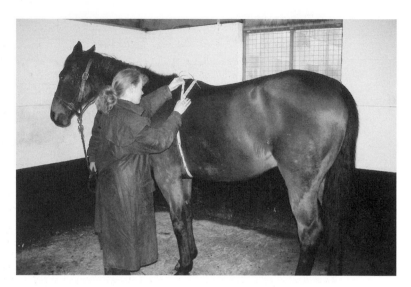

Figure 5.5   Although a weigh pad is the best option a weigh band can be used as a quick and convenient method of monitoring a mare's weight, especially when used in conjunction with assessment of body condition by eye and feel. © CABI.

Assessing body condition is often the best way to gauge whether the mare is being fed correctly and can be assessed by eye and feel. A condition score of 3 should be aimed for throughout pregnancy (Figure 3.10, p. 68).

The nutrition of the lactating mare is considered in Chapter 7 and so this section will concentrate on the non-lactating pregnant mare. The same general ground rules apply to feeding the mare as to any horse. Mares should be fed little and often to ensure that the gut is not overfilled and digestive upsets should be avoided by making any changes to feed gradually. All feed must be of good quality with adequate roughage and ideally all batches of hay, haylage, etc. should be analysed so that a balanced ration can be made up with the addition of concentrates and the correct supplements where necessary. A balanced ration provides protein, energy, vitamins, minerals and water. The relative amounts of these nutrients required depends upon not only the reproductive status of the animal, i.e. pregnant, lactating etc., but also on the individual horse, size, condition, work done and appetite. The relative amounts of nutrients should also be balanced within the diet.

The advised levels of energy (measured as digestible energy or DE), protein (measured as crude protein or CP), lysine (an important amino acid and indicator of protein quality), calcium (Ca) and phosphorus (P) for different weight mares at different stages of pregnancy are given in Tables 5.2 and 5.3. Table 5.2 gives the actual amount of energy, protein, lysine, calcium and phosphorus required by a range of animals on a stud, including the pregnant mare. However, the analysis of a feed is normally given as a percentage of the nutrient within that feed, i.e. most concentrate feeds for late pregnant mares contain 13–15% crude protein (CP). This figure should be printed on the bag of feed. Table 5.3 gives the overall percentage of energy, protein, lysine, calcium and phosphorus that the diet needs to contain to provide the nutrients required as given in Table 5.2. It also gives an indication of the relative amounts of hay and concentrates which need to be fed to meet requirements. When using Table 5.3 to help establish the correct ration for a horse you need to have an idea of the animal's appetite. As a rough guide, a horse will eat 2% of its body weight as dry feed per day, i.e. a 500 kg horse will eat 10 kg of dry feed per day. However, it must be remembered that no feed is 100% dry, it will also contain varying amounts of water which will affect appetite. There is also considerable variation between individuals and especially in late pregnancy when there is a reduction in appetite due to a restriction in the room for the gut. The figure of 2% therefore can only be used as a rough guide.

During early pregnancy the demands on the mare are small, the same as that for maintenance, and she should not gain any significant weight. Her nutrient requirements can, therefore, be met from 100% good quality forage. However, as she progresses into the last 100 days of pregnancy, she should be expected to gain around 0.25 kg/day, as it is during this time that most fetal growth occurs. At this point her feed must be adjusted to provide the extra nutrients she now requires. In general, as pregnancy progresses into the last 100 days, energy and protein intake need to increase. Energy requirement increases by about 10%, the equivalent to a horse in light work. Protein is more critical and increases by about 20%. This increase in protein and energy levels in the last 100 days can in theory be met by feeding more and better quality forage. However, the quality of forage available is rarely good enough, also at this stage the uterus is so big that it begins to limit the capacity of the digestive tract and therefore not enough forage can be eaten to provide the nutrients required. Good-quality, low bulk feeds, which are high in nutrients are needed, such as concentrates. In practice, therefore, most mares in late pregnancy are fed at the most 80% good quality forage and 20% high energy/protein concentrates. Whether these concentrates are one of the many concentrate mixes sold for late pregnant mares or a home-made mix of straights (i.e. raw ingredients such as oats, maize, sugar beet etc.) does not matter, the important thing is that along with the forage fed they meet the mare's requirements (Table 5.2).

Table 5.2 The daily nutrient requirements of different classes of horse of varying weights. Adapted with permission from *Nutrient Requirements of Horses*, Fifth Edn, 1989, National Academy of Sciences, National Academy Press, Washington, D.C.

Animal	Weight (kg)	Mature weight (kg)	Daily gain (kg)	DE (Mcal)	Crude protein (g)	Lysine (g)	Calcium (Ca) (g)	Phosphorus (P) (g)
Maintenance	200	200	0	7.4	296	10	8	6
	500	500	0	16.4	656	23	20	14
	700	700	0	21.3	851	30	28	20
Growing horses								
Weanling 4 months	75	200	0.40	7.3	365	15	16	9
	175	500	0.85	14.4	720	30	34	19
	225	700	1.10	19.7	986	41	44	25
Weanling 6 months Moderate growth	95	200	0.30	7.6	378	16	13	7
	215	500	0.65	15.0	750	32	29	16
	275	700	0.80	20.0	1001	42	37	20
Rapid growth	95	200	0.40	8.7	433	18	17	9
	215	500	0.85	17.2	860	36	36	20
	275	700	1.00	22.2	1111	47	43	24
Yearling 12 months Moderate growth	140	200	0.20	8.7	392	17	12	7
	325	500	0.50	18.9	851	36	29	16
	420	700	0.70	26.1	1176	50	39	22
Rapid growth	140	200	0.30	10.3	462	19	15	8
	325	500	0.65	21.3	956	40	34	19
	420	700	0.85	28.5	1281	54	44	24
Yearling 18 months Not in training	170	200	0.10	8.3	375	16	10	6
	400	500	0.35	19.8	893	38	27	15
	525	700	0.50	27.0	1215	51	37	20
In training	170	200	0.10	11.6	522	22	14	8
	400	500	0.35	26.5	1195	50	36	20
	525	700	0.50	36.0	1615	68	49	27

Two year old 24 months								
Not in training	185	200	0.05	7.9	337	13	9	5
	450	500	0.20	18.8	800	32	24	13
	600	700	0.35	26.3	1117	45	35	19
In training	185	200	0.05	11.4	485	19	13	7
	450	500	0.20	26.3	1117	45	34	19
	600	700	0.35	36.0	1529	61	48	27
Pregnant Mares								
9 months pregnant	200	–	–	8.2	361	13	16	12
	500	–	–	18.2	801	28	35	26
	700	–	–	23.6	1039	36	45	33
10 months pregnant	200	–	–	8.4	368	13	16	12
	500	–	–	18.5	815	29	35	26
	700	–	–	24.0	1058	37	46	34
11 months pregnant	200	–	–	8.9	391	14	17	13
	500	–	–	19.7	866	30	37	28
	700	–	–	25.5	1124	39	49	35
Lactating mare								
Foaling – 3 months	200	–	–	13.7	688	24	27	18
	500	–	–	28.3	1427	50	56	36
	700	–	–	37.9	1997	70	78	51
Weaning – 3 months	200	–	–	12.2	528	18	18	11
	500	–	–	24.3	1048	37	36	22
	700	–	–	32.4	1468	51	50	31
Stallion	200	–	–	9.3	370	13	11	8
	500	–	–	20.5	820	29	25	18
	700	–	–	26.6	1064	37	32	23

Table 5.3 Nutrient concentrations in total diets for different classes of horse of varying weights (100% DM). Values assume a concentrate feed containing 3.3 Mcal/kg and hay containing 2.0 Mcal/kg dry matter. Adapted with permission from *Nutrient Requirements of Horses*, Fifth Edn, 1989, National Academy of Sciences, National Academy Press, Washington, D.C.

Animal	DE (Mcal/kg)	Diet proportions		Crude protein (%)	Lysine (%)	Calcium (Ca) (%)	Phosphorus (P) (%)
		concentrate (%)	hay (%)				
Maintenance	2.00	0	100	8.0	0.28	0.24	0.17
Growing horses							
Weanling 4 months	2.90	70	30	14.5	0.60	0.68	0.38
Weanling 6 months							
Moderate growth	2.90	70	30	14.5	0.61	0.56	0.31
Rapid growth	2.90	70	30	14.5	0.61	0.61	0.34
Yearling 12 months							
Moderate growth	2.80	60	40	12.6	0.53	0.43	0.24
Rapid growth	2.80	60	40	12.6	0.53	0.45	0.25
Yearling 18 months							
Not in training	2.50	45	55	11.3	0.48	0.34	0.19
In training	2.65	50	50	12.0	0.50	0.36	0.20
Two year old 24 months							
Not in training	2.45	35	65	10.4	0.42	0.31	0.17
In training	2.65	50	50	11.3	0.45	0.34	0.20
Pregnant mare							
9 months	2.25	20	80	10.0	0.35	0.43	0.32
10 months	2.25	20	80	10.0	0.35	0.43	0.32
11 months	2.40	30	70	10.6	0.37	0.45	0.34
Lactating mare							
Foaling – 3 months	2.60	50	50	13.2	0.46	0.52	0.34
Weaning – 3 months	2.45	35	65	11.0	0.37	0.36	0.22
Stallion	2.40	30	70	9.6	0.34	0.29	0.21

Vitamins and minerals are also important, in particular calcium and phosphorus. The calcium:phosphorus ratio is of special importance as both minerals are involved in bone growth. In the pregnant mare not only are they important to the mare herself but also to the fetus. Calcium and phosphorus are normally stored within the bone, much of which is a temporary store and can be used if required, for example if the pregnant mare's diet is low in calcium or phosphorus. However, if this is occurs then her bones will suffer, becoming brittle and possibly unable to take the strain of the increased weight in late pregnancy or the stresses of parturition. The foals of such mares can also suffer from deformities in tissue and bone growth and be generally ill thrifty at birth. As with energy and protein, the time of greatest demand is during the last 100 days of pregnancy when requirements for calcium increase by about 75% and those for phosphorus by about 80% (Table 5.2). Mares in late pregnancy require a diet with 0.43–0.45% calcium and 0.32–0.34% phosphorus (Table 5.3). Most forages fed to horses do not contain these levels of calcium and phosphorus. This combined with the restriction to appetite by the growing fetus means that calcium and phosphorus invariably need to be supplemented in late pregnancy using either a commercial vitamin and mineral supplement or more commonly by using a concentrate feed, which will also help meet the higher energy and protein requirements. Other minerals and vitamins are also important. In the pregnant mare vitamin A is the most important vitamin and deficiency may be linked to foal limb deformities. The mare's requirement again increases in the last 100 days of pregnancy which for mares at pasture can be satisfied by fresh green forage. For mares with little if any access to pasture vitamin A needs to be supplemented.

Finally, water is an often overlooked but vitally important component of any diet. The pregnant mare requires approximately 50 litres/day of water, which must be clean, fresh and available at all times.

In spite of being fed a theoretically perfect ration, the mare's body condition may still indicate that she is being over- or under-fed, if this is the case the ration must be changed accordingly.

5.5.3 Parasite control

Parasite control is of significant importance. A high parasite count is often the reason why some animals appear as 'poor doers', and parasites cause a large quantity of the food to be wasted. If the worm burden is excessive, damage to the gastrointestinal tract may be permanent, condemning the mare to being a 'bad doer' for the rest of her life and may even be the cause of death. Ascarids and threadworms are the main parasites associated with disease in foals; ascarids, large strongyles (redworm), small strongyles, bots, tapeworm, lungworm and pinworms are the main parasites for animals up to three years of age; whereas large strongyles (redworm), small strongyles, bots, tapeworm, lungworm and pinworm are the main parasites of adult horses. There are numerous wormers (anthelmintics) on the market and they all have a different range of species that they are effective against, as well as different effects on different stages of parasite development (adults or larvae) and different dosing frequencies. These wormers all fall into one of three families: avermectins; pyrimidines; and benzimidazoles (Table 5.4). Correct use of anthelmintics is essential for the health of all stock. Traditionally it has been advised that all horses should be wormed every six weeks throughout the year. It is now known that worming need not be so frequent during winter if the temperature is below freezing, and that strategic worming of only those horses with a high faecal worm count, along with good rotational grazing management and dung removal can be just as effective.

Table 5.4 Common parasites of the horse and anthelmintics active against them.

Parasite	Family of drug/wormer	Active ingredient
Adult large strongyles (redworm), small strongyles, pinworms	Benzimidazoles	Fenbendazole
	–	Mebendazole
	–	Oxfendazole
	–	Thiabendazole
	Avermectins	Ivermectin
	Pyrimidines	Pyrantel
Larvae large strongyles (redworm), small strongyles	Benzimidazoles	Fenbendazole
	–	Oxfendazole
	Avermectins	Iermectin
	–	Moxidectin
Threadworms (*Strongyloides westeri*)	Benzimidazoles	Thiabendazole
	–	Fenbendazole
	Avermectins	Ivermectin
Ascarids	Avermectins	Ivermectin
	Benzimidazoles	Fenbendazole
	–	Oxfendazole
	–	Mebendazole
	Pyrimidines	Pyrantel
Lungworm	Avermectin	Ivermectin
	Benzimidazoles	Fenbendazole
	–	Mebendazole
Bots	Avermectin	Ivermectin
Tapeworm	Pyrimidines	Pyrantel

Whatever system is used, rotation of wormers between the three different families within a period of twelve months is essential to avoid parasites developing resistance to anthelmintics. For this reason confining the use of anthelmintics to carriers and specific times of the year is increasingly practised today. In recent years it has become apparent that small strongyles are increasingly resistant to wormers in the benzimidazole group, although fortunately wormers in the avermectin group are still effective.

As an adult animal the pregnant mare is susceptible to large and small strongyles, bots, tapeworm, lungworm and pinworm. Foals are particularly susceptible to ascarids and threadworms and so wormers against these are particularly important to prevent infestation of the foal. Anthelmintics within all three of the families are effective against a range of these parasites (Table 5.4) and so the appropriate ones should be selected for use. However, care must be taken in worming pregnant mares since not all wormers are suitable – advice must be sought. In general, it is recommended that no wormers be used in the last month of pregnancy due to the possible risk of inducing premature birth. Some studs however worm all mares immediately before parturition to ensure that the foal is not exposed to a high parasite burden at birth.

5.5.4 Vaccinations

The vaccination programme required by a mare depends on the diseases present in the country in which she lives. In many European countries and the USA, vaccination against tetanus and influenza is automatic, proof of vaccination is nearly always required before a mare will be accepted onto a stud. Annual boosters of influenza and tetanus vaccination should be given four to six weeks before parturition to ensure that the mare's body raises enough antibodies to pass to the colostrum, ready for the foal.

Equine rhinopneumonitis (equine herpesvirus type 1 (EHV 1)) is a problem in the USA and is becoming increasingly so in the UK. This infection causes abortion, normally in the last third of pregnancy, in up to 70% of infected mares. If an outbreak is suspected, or routine protection is required, vaccination can be given in months five, seven and nine of pregnancy.

Equine viral arteritis (EVA) also causes abortion and a vaccine is now available. Although EVA is a problem in parts of Europe and USA, it is not common at present in the UK, but complacency cannot be allowed. Vaccination is available and may be given to pregnant mares, but not in the last two months of pregnancy. Testing for and certification to prove disease-free status is often required by studs prior to a mare's arrival (Sections 3.4.1, p. 69 and 3.5.1, p. 76). The Horse Race Betting Levy Board (HRBLB) annual codes of practice give advice on both EHV and EVA.

In other parts of the world routine vaccination for eastern and western equine encephalomyelitis, equine pneumonitis (EHV 4), rabies and potomac horse fever may be considered. With the exception of rabies, all vaccinations can be given in the last four weeks of pregnancy to give protection to the foal via colostrum. Vaccination for strangles, botulism, anthrax, salmonella typhimurium and leptospirosis is possible but only advised in areas of risk.

5.5.5 Teeth and feet care

The teeth of the pregnant mare should not be neglected. Regular teeth rasping ensures that all the plates are level and can efficiently grind food, which helps digestion and maximises the nutrients obtained. This is of greatest importance when the mare's system is under stress with a high demand for nutrients, such as in late pregnancy.

The majority of brood mares are unshod; even so regular hoof trimming should be carried out. Poor feet cause pain, and this pain can be made worse by the weight of late pregnancy. Such mares will be reluctant to exercise, resulting in the problems previously discussed (Section 5.5.1, p. 120). Some mares are turned out to stud with muscle or bone problems so may need orthopaedic shoeing, especially in late pregnancy. Shod mares must however have shoes removed prior to parturition to prevent damage to the foal.

5.6 ABORTION

Abortion in the mare is always tragic, although in many cases it is nature's way of removing a fetus which would never have survived. It has several causes, many of which cannot be avoided, but some may be preventable with good management. The major causes of abortion are: multiple pregnancies, physical abnormalities, infection, genetic abnormalities, hormonal abnormalities and stress.

5.6.1 Multiple pregnancies

Multiple pregnancies are the single most significant cause of non-infectious abortion in the mare. The mare's uterus is unable to carry more than one pregnancy successfully to term and so multiple pregnancies have a high chance of aborting if left untreated (Sections 1.4.3.1, p. 29 and 5.4, p. 119).

5.6.2 Physical abnormalities

There are a range of different physical abnormalities which may cause abortion. Many are associated with older mares and especially those which have been pregnant many times before (multiparous). Multiparous older mares tend to ovulate less viable ova which, if fertilised, often abort in early pregnancy. The endometrium of such mares also suffers from wear and tear from the numerous previous pregnancies (chronic non-infective endometritis) and so provides a less effective attachment for the placenta. Older mares also have a higher incidence of uterine cysts and adhesions, all of which disrupt placental attachment. The endometrium of some mares may be under or over developed due to a genetic defect, age, failure to recover from the last pregnancy (delayed uterine involution see Section 7.6.2, p. 183), adverse reaction to semen after covering etc., all of these also affect the ability of the uterus to maintain another pregnancy.

5.6.3 Infectious abortion

Infections can be bacterial, viral or fungal. All these infections cause endometritis (inflammation of the endometrium) which, depending upon when the infection occurs, will either prevent the pregnancy developing during the early stages (early embryonic death, EED) or if later in pregnancy will cause placentitis (infection of the placenta) and late abortion. The most common causes of infectious abortion are bacterial and may cause abortion at any time during pregnancy. The bacteria involved are usually the bacteria which cause venereal disease (*Taylorella equigenitalis, Pseudomonas aeruginosa, Klebsiella pneumoniae*) or bacteria generally found in the environment (*E. coli, Streptococcus zooepidemicus, Staphylococcus aureus*). Many of these bacteria must be tested for before mares will be accepted for covering (HRBLB *Code of Practice*, see Sections 3.4.1, p. 69 and 3.5.1, p. 76).

Viral infections are less common and tend to cause abortion in late pregnancy. The two most worthy of note are, equine viral arteritis (EVA) and equine herpesvirus-1 (EHV 1). EVA is spread from horse to horse via close contact through respiration, at covering or via infected placenta. It is uncommon in the UK but is evident in other parts of the world; vaccination may be advised and is successful (Section 5.5.4, p. 129). EHV 1 can again be transferred via respiration, placental material, soiled bedding and is found in semen. The virus causes the placenta to separate from the endometrium causing the fetus to suffocate, die and abort usually in the last four months.

Fungal infections are uncommon, of those seen *Candida albicans*, a yeast, is most common. Fungal infections can cause pregnancies to

Managing Your Mare at Foaling 6

6.1 INTRODUCTION

Foaling your mare (parturition) is the most exciting part of breeding but is potentially the most dangerous for both mare and foal. Average pregnancy (gestation) length in the thoroughbred-type mare is 320–335 days, ponies tend to give birth about two weeks earlier. Parturition is the active expulsion of the fetus, along with associated fluids and placenta by contractions of the uterine muscles.

6.2 MANAGING YOUR MARE AS FOALING APPROACHES

Approximately six weeks before the mare's expected delivery date, she should be brought onto the foaling unit or the yard at which she is to foal. This begins the gradual process of familiarising the mare with the surroundings in which she will foal and be kept immediately after foaling. This will allow her to become accustomed to management practices, especially if she is to foal away from home, as well as to changes in feed, exercise, housing and routine.

If the mare is foaling away from home, a period of six weeks is also required to allow her immune system to raise the necessary antibodies to any bacteria in her new foaling environment. This will not only give the mare protection, but also allow enough time for the antibodies to pass to the colostrum and so be available to the foal to give it immediate protection after suckling. It is therefore advisable to vaccinate mares during this six week period (Section 5.5.4, p. 129).

Exercise is very important. Regular free exercise in a paddock or field will be adequate for most mares and will help maintain fitness for foaling as well as reduce the chances of fluid retention in the legs. A slightly laxative diet, by including bran in the feed, may be given in the last week or so as many mares suffer from constipation in late pregnancy, especially if exercise is limited. Lastly, but by no means least, clean, fresh water must be available at all times.

Throughout the preparation of the mare for foaling, the mare should be observed for the characteristic signs of imminent parturition.

6.2.1 Signs of imminent parturition

There are several signs which indicate that your mare is about to foal, these can be seen at any time from around the last three weeks of pregnancy. Not all mares show all these signs, so a combination of the following signs should be looked for, they should be adequate to give warning of parturition and allow preparations to be made.

Changes in the appearance of the udder are one of the first signs that parturition is approaching. During the last month milk production starts, the udder increases in size as colostrum is produced and stored. The udder may feel warm to touch, and swollen with milk (Figure 6.1).

As the udder fills, the bases of the teats stretch and the teats appear to shorten, but as milk production increases they fill with milk becoming longer and tender to touch. Some mares may start to lose milk as production gets too great for the udder's storage capacity and the sphincter at the end of the teat can no longer stop milk leaking. If a mare does start to lose milk this can be a problem as this is in fact valuable colostrum. A mare only produces a set amount of colostrum and will produce no more once the initial amount has been lost. It is therefore very important to collect this leaked milk into a sterile container

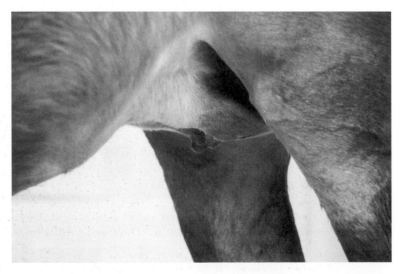

Figure 6.1 The udder of a mare five days before foaling. © CABI.

and freeze it ready for thawing and feeding to the foal immediately after birth. Colostrum can be safely frozen from one year to the next. Many mares 'wax up', a term given to the clotting of this colostrum at the end of the teat (Figure 6.2). This is a good sign of imminent parturition. However, if wax is not seen, this does not necessarily mean that parturition is not close as these plugs of colostrum can easily become dislodged, especially when mares are turned out.

The concentration of several minerals, including calcium, in mammary gland secretions changes as parturition approaches. Water hardener strips can be used to indicate an increase in calcium concentrations and so warn of approaching parturition.

Changes in the birth canal may also be seen as parturition approaches. In the last three weeks a hollowness may appear on either side of the tail root as the muscles and ligaments in the pelvic area relax. The whole area may appear to sink with this relaxation which eases the foal's passage through the birth canal (Figure 6.3). In late pregnancy as the fetus increases in size, the abdomen expands becoming characteristically large and pendulous. However, in the final stages of pregnancy the abdomen appears to shrink as the foal moves up into the birth canal (Figure 6.4).

As parturition becomes imminent, the mare may become restless and agitated, especially as first stage labour starts. In the wild, at this stage, the mare would move away from the herd to find a quiet area, and this is why some housed mares become quite agitated and show 'nesting-like' behaviour such as kicking up and redistributing their

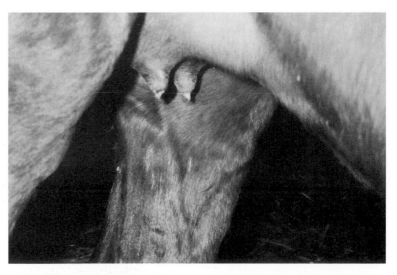

Figure 6.2 One of the signs of imminent foaling is the accumulation of dried colostrum on the teats of the mare, known as 'waxing up'. Dried colostrum may also be seen on the inside of the hind legs. © CABI.

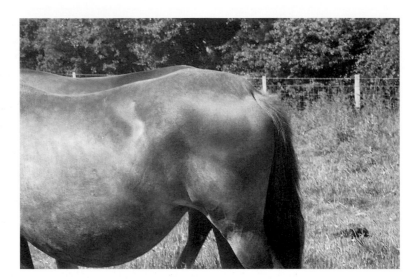

Figure 6.3 A further sign of imminent parturition is a hollowing of the back above the pelvis and either side of the tail, as a result of a relaxation of the birth canal. © CABI.

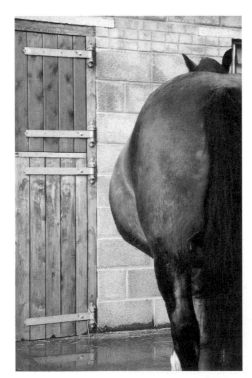

Figure 6.4 One of the obvious signs of pregnancy is a large pendulous abdomen. However, immediately prior to parturition the abdomen appears to shrink as the foal moves up into the birth canal.

bed, pacing the box etc. As the mare moves into first stage labour her body temperature will increase and she may sweat profusely, internally her cervix will start to dilate and she may show signs similar to colic, e.g. walking in circles, swishing her tail, looking around at her sides, kicking her abdomen etc.

Many commercial products have been produced to try to predict the timing of parturition, particularly aimed at big studs with many valuable mares. These make use of some of the mare's natural signals, reacting to the movement of the mare, or measuring any increase in body temperature or sweating, stretching of the vulval lips etc. Once triggered these products normally produce a signal which is transmitted to a buzzer or equivalent at a distance. None of these products is ideal and they often give false alarms, because of this closed circuit television is widely used, allowing observation but from a distance and in relative comfort.

As soon as the mare shows any of the signs of being close to parturition she should be moved to her foaling box or to a small paddock.

6.2.2 Foaling facilities

A mare may foal either in a specially built foaling unit or outside. Most thoroughbred-type mares and those of significant value, especially if foaling early in the season as well as maiden or difficult mares, are foaled indoors. Late foalers and the native-type mares are often foaled outdoors. Indoor foaling allows more control and easier monitoring and protection from the weather, but it runs a higher risk of infection unless the foaling boxes are kept scrupulously clean. Outdoor foaling is harder to monitor but is closer to the natural environment and tends to run a lower infection risk, and is increasingly popular. Whichever system is chosen, the stages of labour and their management are very similar.

6.2.2.1 Foaling box

If your mare is to foal inside, a foaling box will be required; this should be at least $5\,m^2$ with good ventilation, but should be draught free. The box required is larger than normal as most mares foal lying down so they need space to stretch out. Traditionally, the floor covering is a deep bed of straw, which provides a soft, warm, dust-free surface onto which the foal can be born and is still used by many studs (Figure 6.8 (a), p. 145). More recently, rubber matting has become increasingly popular which, though expensive, provides a clean, insulated and dust-free floor which can be washed and disinfected easily. A small straw bed is also sometimes used as it is perceived to be warmer. Beds made from paper and wood shavings are not advised as they tend to stick to the newborn foal and are unpleasant for the mare when she licks the foal.

The foaling box should be free of any protrusions which may cause damage to the mare or foal. Ideally, it should have rounded corners to reduce the risk of the mare getting cast. Hay nets should not be used as the foal can get itself caught up in them, ideally hay should be fed from the ground. High hayracks avoid the wastage of feeding off the floor but run the risk of seeds getting into the mare's and foal's eyes and ears. In an ideal unit each box would have two doors, one to the outside for horse access and another facing into a central sitting area for access for helpers and viewing. A radiant heat lamp for use with weak foals is also a good idea.

Once the mare has settled into her foaling quarters it is a case of careful watching and waiting from some distance. Disturbance should be avoided, although careful observation is essential as it can minimise the time from the first signs of trouble to action and can be crucial in saving lives.

6.2.2.2 Foaling kit

In readiness for foaling the following equipment should be organised:

- Telephone number of your vet – the vet should have been warned beforehand
- Mare halter and lead rope
- Towels
- Bucket
- Soap or antibacterial wash
- Cotton wool
- Access to warm water
- Obstetric lubricant
- Obstetric ropes
- Sharp knife or scalpel
- Radiant heat lamp
- Antiseptic spray/navel dressing
- Feeding bottles for milk/colostrum
- Gastrointestinal feeding tube
- Access to colostrum e.g. frozen colostrum

6.3 MANAGEMENT OF FOALING

Parturition is divided into three stages; stage 1, the positioning of the foal into the birth canal; stage 2, the birth of the foal; and stage 3, the expulsion of the placenta. All three stages are caused by strong contractions of the uterine muscle (myometrium), with some involvement of the abdominal muscles.

6.3.1 First stage of labour

Stage one involves a gradual build up of uterine muscle contractions and normally lasts between one and four hours, though some mares show signs of going in and out of first stage labour for several hours. The contractions push the foal up into the birth canal (Figure 6.5).

The uterine muscle contractions start as mild waves which move from the tip of the uterine horn towards the cervix. These contractions, helped by the movement of the mare and, to a certain extent, by those of the foal, move the foal into the birth canal. Throughout late pregnancy the foal lies in a curled-up position (its vertebrae lying along the line of the mother's abdomen). During first stage labour the foal turns over into an extended position with its forelimbs, head and neck fully stretched out (Figure 6.6).

Together with the changes in the position of the foal, the cervix gradually dilates, the vulva continues to relax and secretions appear. At the end of stage one the fetus's forelegs and muzzle push their way through the dilating cervix, encouraging further dilation and taking with them the placenta. At the cervix, the placenta is particularly thin and not attached to the cervix (this part of the placenta is known as the *cervical star*) this area ruptures as the pressure of the muscle contractions against the placental fluids builds up, forcing them and the

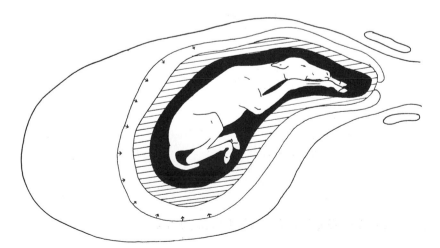

Figure 6.5 The forces which cause the onset of the first stage of labour are provided by contractions of the uterine muscle, as indicated by the arrows. © CABI.

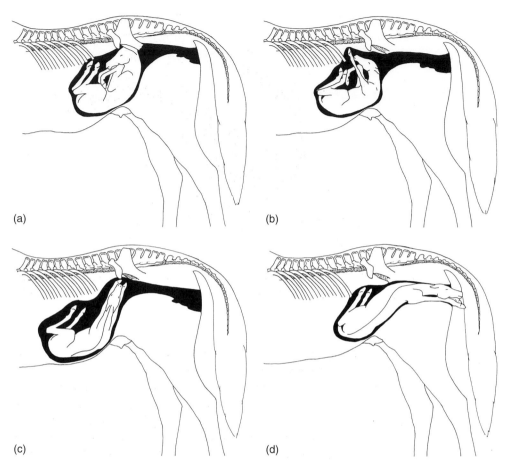

(a)

(b)

(c)

(d)

Figure 6.6 During the first stage of labour the foal gradually turns and extends within the birth canal ready to be pushed out by the contractions of second-stage labour. © CABI.

fetus through the cervix. The rupture of the placenta causes a release of the allantoic fluid (breaking of the waters) and is the signal for the beginning of the second stage of labour.

During the first stage of labour the mare will seem restless and may repeatedly get up and lie down. She may well sweat profusely and appear uneasy, glancing at her flanks and grimacing, showing signs similar to colic. This continual moving around is thought to help position the foal within the birth canal and excessive rolling may be the first sign that the foal is incorrectly positioned. It is difficult to state how long first stage labour should last and at what stage you should call for assistance, as some mares will show several false starts in the days before birth. However, as a general rule, the veterinary surgeon should be called if the mare seems to be in discomfort for a long time,

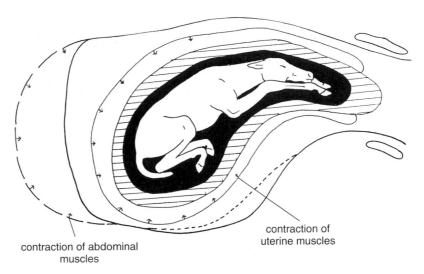

Figure 6.7 The second stage of labour involves stronger contractions of the uterine muscle helped by contractions of the abdominal muscles, as indicated by the arrows. © CABI.

appears very agitated and sweats profusely, and before she is in any danger of becoming exhausted. During stage one she requires no special attention except to be closely watched for possible problems and for the onset of the second stage. Once the mare is in first stage labour, her tail should be bandaged, the perineal area thoroughly washed and if she has had a Caslick's operation she should be cut (undergo an episiotomy) (Figure 6.8 (b), p. 145). Some mares may lose milk prior to, or during, the first stage of delivery and this should be collected to be fed to the foal (Section 6.2.1, p. 136, Figure 6.2, p. 137).

6.3.2 Second stage of labour

Stage two marks the beginning of very strong uterine muscle contractions. The reduction in pressure within the uterus which results from the release of allantoic fluid at the end of stage one seems to be the trigger for these strong contractions. The fluid released also lubricates the vagina to ease the foal's passage. The contractions continue in a wave-like fashion from the tips of the uterine horn to the cervix but in stage two are helped by contractions of the abdominal muscles (Figure 6.7), called voluntary straining. This is brought about by the mare breathing in deeply which depresses the diaphragm, increasing the pressure in the abdomen, which in turn increases the pressure on the uterus and also causes the abdominal muscles themselves to contract in response to the pressure. The contraction of the abdominal muscles further increases pressure on the uterus which helps to push out the foal. Voluntary straining is most efficient if the mare is lying down, and this is why most mares give birth lying down.

These strong contractions continue until the birth of the foal. At the start of stage two the amniotic sac is often visible bulging through the vulva (Figure 6.8 (c)) and within it should be felt the foal's forelegs and muzzle (Figure 6.8 (d)). The foal is delivered forelegs first with its head between its legs (Figures 6.8 (e) and (f)). Once the shoulders and thorax of the foal have passed through the birth canal the remainder of the foal passes relatively easily (Figure 6.8 (g)). The shape of the birth canal is curved and so the foal is born with its head down towards the mare's hind legs. It is important to remember this if you are aiding parturition by pulling a foal. At the end of stage two the foal lies with its hind limbs still within the mare, the mare can then lean round to lick it (Figure 6.8 (h)).

The management of second-stage labour is more important than first-stage labour, but again normally involves watching from a discrete distance with interference only if a problem is identified. Within five minutes of the start of second-stage labour many studs will carry out a brief internal examination to ensure that the foal is presented correctly (Figure 6.8 (d)). If all is well the mare should be left alone to deliver naturally, however, if the foal is not presented correctly help should now be called. Second-stage labour should last on average 15 minutes (range 5–30 minutes).

Figure 6.8 (a)–(p) Parturition in the mare: (a) most mares will lie down to give birth, straw is a good foaling bed; (b) if the mare has had a Caslick's operation she should have it cut (episiotomy) at the start of stage one; (c) at the beginning of stage two the amniotic sac may be seen as a white membrane protruding through the mare's vulva; (d) at this stage a brief internal examination may be done to check if the position of the foal is correct; (e) one foot and then (f) both feet and head should be seen in the amniotic sac, with one foot slightly in front of the other; (g) once the hips are through the birth canal the hard work is over, note that the foal is delivered in a curved manner, down towards the mare's hind legs; (h) at the end of stage two the foal may lie for some time with its hind legs still within the vagina of the mare; (i) if the amnion is still around the foal's head it should be removed immediately to allow it to breathe; (j) the foal will be born still attached to the placenta, which is inside the mare, by the umbilical cord. The cord should not be cut but allowed to break naturally when the mare or foal moves; (k) soon after birth the healthy foal should be in a sitting up position; (l) the foal may be dried off and at the same time the heart rate checked, care must be taken to allow the mare time to lick the foal; (m) the placenta should be tied up to prevent the mare (n) standing on it and tearing it; (o) third stage labour expels the placenta (in the foreground of the photograph) which should be examined for completeness, the white amniotic sac is shown in the background; (p) the placenta is expelled inside out. The red, velvety outer surface of the placenta which was attached to the uterus being on the inside with the smooth inner surface of the placenta on the outside. (Photographs Rufus Stephen, © CABI.)

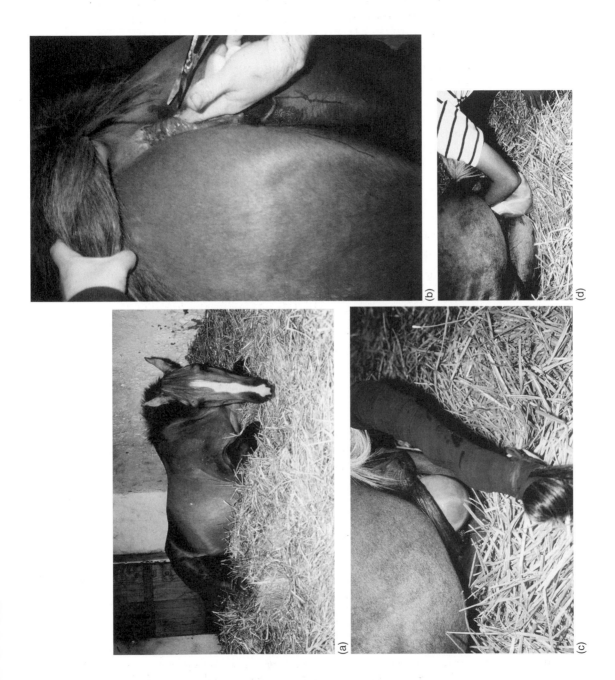

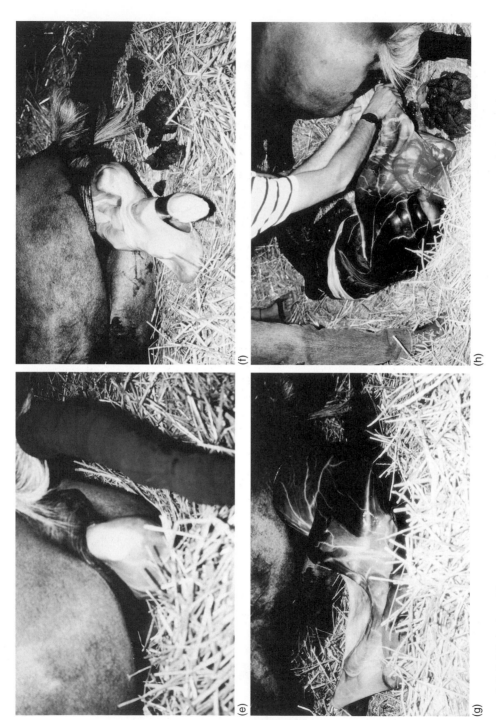

Figure 6.8 (a)–(p) (cont'd)

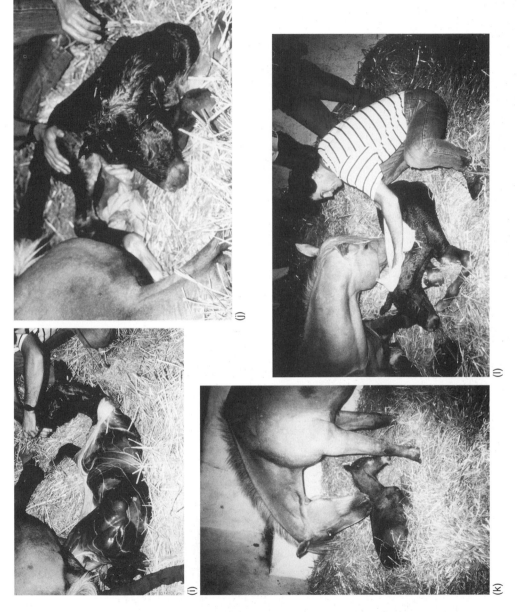

Figure 6.8 (a)–(p) *(cont'd)*

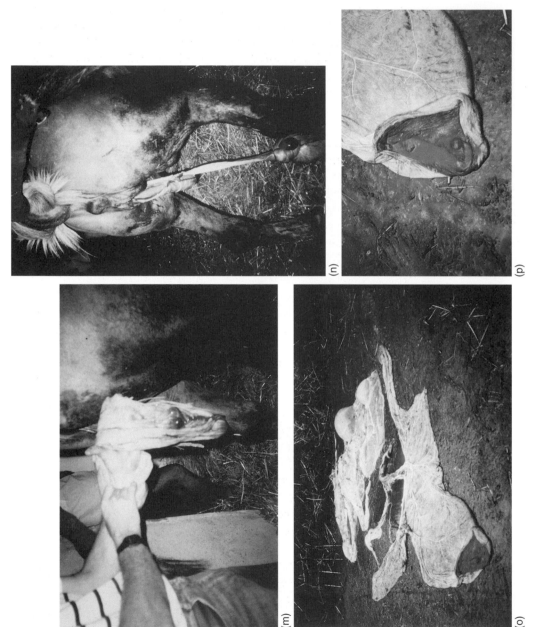

Figure 6.8 (a)–(p) *(cont'd)*

6.3.3 Management immediately after foaling

Immediately after birth, if the foal shows signs of distress or is limp or weak, the amniotic sac should be broken immediately and the foal's head lifted to help breathing (Figure 6.8 (i)). The foal should be left with its hind legs within its mother and the umbilical cord intact (Figures 6.8 (i) and (j)). The umbilical cord will naturally shrivel up and break, forming a seal about 3 cm from the foal's abdomen, when either the mare or foal moves. Breaking the umbilical cord early risks the foal losing up to 1.5 litres of blood which would normally drain into it from the placenta. The foal's legs within the vulva appear to have a tranquillising effect on the mare, and most mares are reluctant to get up immediately, though they will turn to lick the foal. A mare may lie down for up to 30 minutes, providing she is sitting up and interested in the foal, this should be encouraged as it allows the reproductive tract time to contract and so reduces the passage of air and bacteria into the uterus through the relaxed vulva when she moves. Any such contamination increases the chance of endometritis and delays when the mare can be covered again (Section 7.6.2, p. 183). Temporary clips can be used after stage three to close the upper lips of the vulva to reduce the passage of air into the uterus. These clips can easily be removed two to three days after foaling at the normal post-foaling internal examination and if necessary replaced by a Caslick's operation.

This period of time immediately after birth marks the beginning of maternal foal bonding and recognition. The mare–foal bond can be irretrievably damaged by interference, however well intentioned, so care should be taken at this stage. A mare which damages her newborn foal is a very rare occurence but it can be the result of her being disturbed or stressed by unnecessary human interference. Mares may nibble or gently bite their foals to encourage them to move (Figure 6.8 (k)) but too much aggression may require the mare to be muzzled. Very occasionally mares, usually maiden, kick or attack their foals so require tranquillising for a short period of time. Tranquillisers may also be used to calm a mare so that the foal can suckle.

Immediately after delivery the foal can be dried off (Figure 6.8 (l)) and the broken umbilical cord dressed with an antiseptic spray or dip, such as very dilute iodine or chlorohexidine to prevent infection. At this stage the foal's heart rate may also be checked by placing a hand on the thorax. Foals used routinely to be given an enema soon after birth, however, this is now thought not to be necessary unless the foal shows signs of meconium retention after 24 hours (Sections 7.2.8, p. 167 and 7.5.1.4, p. 179). Weak foals may require tubing or bottle feeding with colostrum to ensure they get sufficient antibodies as soon as possible after birth. Details of the milestones that a foal should achieve at set times after birth are given in Section 7.2, p. 161.

If you are going to imprint train your foal you should start some time during these first three hours. Imprint training is the rapid introduction of the foal to many of the stimuli or unusual techniques that it will come across in life, e.g. grooming, feet care, clipping, rectal palpation, etc. The idea being that the foal will be happy to accept such stimuli at this stage and so when they are introduced at a later age it will be happy to accept them again.

The mare should be given a feed about an hour after the birth. A light, easily digested and slightly laxative feed is best, plus fresh, good quality forage. Water should initially be given under supervision, unless automatic water feeders are available, to avoid the risk of the foal drowning in a bucket.

6.3.4 Third stage of labour

Uterine contractions continue in stage three but are less intense and are similar to those of stage one. At the same time the placenta begins to shrink away from the uterine endometrium as blood in it drains away towards the foal. This releases the remaining attachment between the placenta and the uterus and forces the placenta to be expelled, inside out, i.e. the placenta is delivered with its red velvety outer surface innermost and the smooth inner surface outermost (Figures 6.8 (o) and (p)). The contractions of third stage labour also help to expel any remaining fluids and help the uterus to return to its pre-pregnancy state (this process is known as *uterine involution*).

Stage three of labour is normally completed within three hours of the end of stage two. During this stage the mare will again appear restless, with behaviour similar to that of stage one. Occasionally, the placenta may be expelled immediately after or at the same time as the foal. At the other extreme it may take several hours. If the placenta is not expelled completely before the mare stands it may be tied up to prevent the mare standing on it and ripping it (Figures 6.8 (m) and (n)). The extra weight provided by the tied-up placenta also encourages expulsion. If completion of third stage labour is delayed for longer than 10 hours this indicates a problem, such as retained placenta (Section 6.4.3.7, p. 159).

As soon as the placenta is expelled, it should be examined for completeness (Figure 6.8 (o)). An effective method of detecting holes and, therefore, any missing fragments, is to tie off both uterine horn ends of the placenta and fill it with water through the cervical star. If there is a leak the break should be examined to ensure that the membranes all fit together and there are no bits missing. If pieces are missing the placenta should be kept and the veterinary surgeon called. Placental retention, even of just a fragment, can lead to septicaemia, laminitis and eventual death if not treated as a matter of urgency (Section 6.4.3.7, p. 159).

6.4 FOALING ABNORMALITIES

Foaling abnormalities also known as dystocia, refer to complications which occur at parturition which prevent a natural birth. They can be divided into fetal dystocia, caused by fetal complications, or maternal dystocia, caused by maternal problems. Dystocia normally causes a delay in birth which may reduce the oxygen supply to the foal, which in turn can cause irreversible problems, particularly brain damage. In many cases of dystocia, changing the foal's position (*mutation*) followed by pulling the foal (*traction*) is all that is required to remedy the problem. Occasionally, more extreme measures such as a Caesarean section or fetotomy (dividing a dead fetus up in the uterus in order to save the mare) are required.

6.4.1 Fetal dystocia

Fetal dystocia is caused almost always by incorrect positioning of the foal (*fetal malpresentations*) making natural birth impossible. Uterine contractions are extremely strong and it takes skill and strength to change the position of the foal. Experienced help is needed. Forward positions are the most common and many can be corrected by pushing the foal back into the uterus, correcting its position, followed by pulling the foal (Figures 6.9–6.12). In addition, there are more complicated forward positions requiring considerable manipulation (Figures 6.13–6.15) with veterinary assistance and which may require a Caesarean section to be performed.

Backward positions may also been seen with the back legs and tail felt within the vagina. In theory the foal can be born in this position but it should be pulled in order to speed up the birth and so reduce the risk of the umbilical cord becoming trapped between the foal's abdomen and the mare's pelvis so starving the foal of oxygen. There is also the danger that the foal may drown by breathing in allantoic fluid. A more complicated backward position may be seen when only

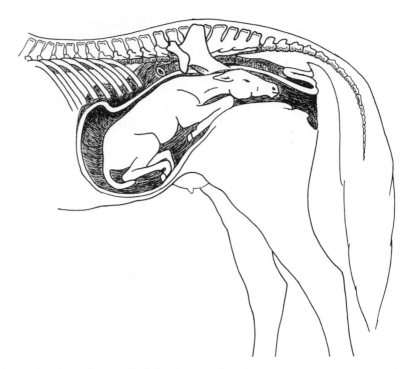

Figure 6.9 Flexion (bending) of one or both forelegs significantly increases the cross-section of the foal making its passage through the birth canal very difficult. © CABI.

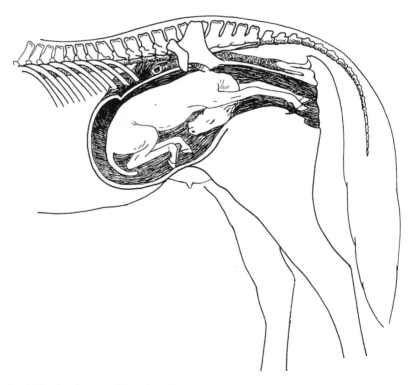

Figure 6.10 If only the forefeet are felt within the vagina, the head may be bent back, again presenting such a wide cross-section of the foal that it is very difficult for the mare to foal naturally. © CABI.

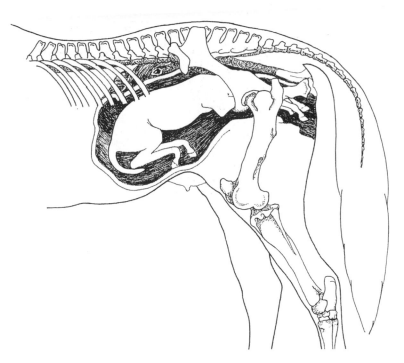

Figure 6.11 If the legs are not fully extended, one or both of the elbows may be bent and become lodged behind the pelvis. © CABI.

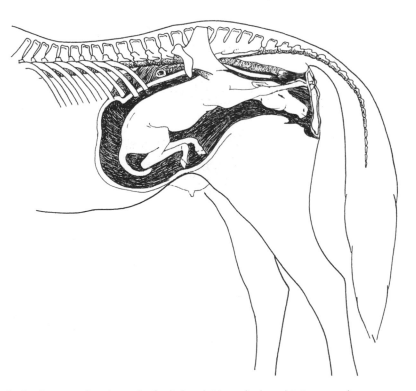

Figure 6.12 The forelegs may be above the foal's head. Not only does this increase the cross-sectional diameter of the foal but there is also the risk of the feet going through the top of the vagina and into the rectum, opening up a rectal vaginal fissure (Section 6.4.3.5, p. 158). © CABI.

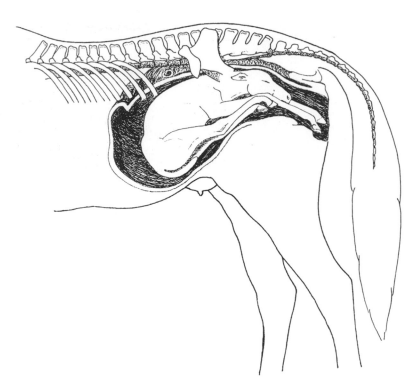

Figure 6.13 If both forefeet and hind feet are felt within the birth canal, veterinary assistance should be called immediately as this position can prove very difficult to correct, especially if the mare has progressed far into labour. © CABI.

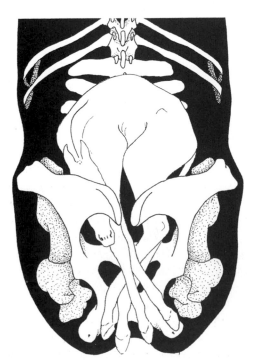

Figure 6.14 A cross-wise presentation also presents four feet first. This can, in theory, be corrected by pushing the hind legs back into the uterus but is very difficult in practice. © CABI.

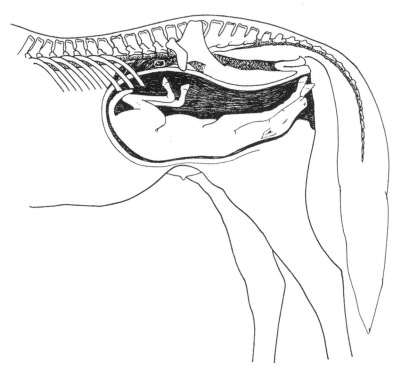

Figure 6.15 In this figure the foal is presented in ventral position. The foal must be turned over into a normal position before delivery is possible. © CABI.

the tail and rump can be felt. This position is known as a breech and veterinary assistance will be required (Figure 6.16).

6.4.2 Maternal dystocia

Maternal dystocia is the failure of natural delivery due to a problem with the mare. Most conditions are rare but one of the more common is placenta previa. This is when the intact red placenta appears through the mare's vulva because it has failed to rupture at the cervical star. This may be simply due to extra thick placental membranes, but could be due to rupture elsewhere which will result in the early separation of the placenta from the uterus and, therefore, in oxygen starvation in the foal. Whatever the cause, as soon as the placenta is seen, the membranes should be cut. Foaling will then usually progress normally although the foal should be watched carefully for signs of brain damage. Some mares have small pelvic openings as a result of an accident or fracture or malnutrition in early life. In

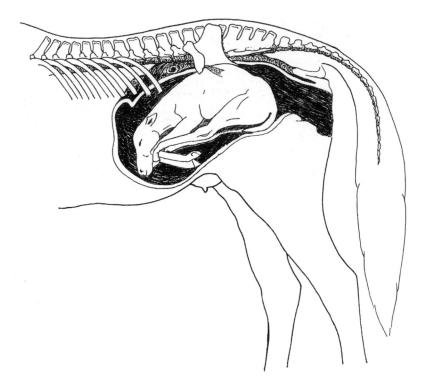

Figure 6.16 If only the tail and rump of the foal are felt within the vagina, this is a true breech position and will require veterinary assistance. © CABI.

such cases a Caesarean section is often required and such mares should not be bred again. Conditions such as *uterine torsion* (twist) and *uterine inertia* (exhaustion) may also occur and require veterinary assistance.

6.4.3 Abnormal conditions

Abnormal conditions associated with parturition do not normally directly prevent delivery but cause concern for the well-being of the mare and foal. These conditions may occur before, during or after labour. They are most commonly seen in older, multiparous mares and those which have suffered from problems in the past.

6.4.3.1 Ruptured pre-pubic tendon

The pre-pubic tendon is attached to, and supports, the abdominal muscles. Accident or old age can cause it to rupture under the strain

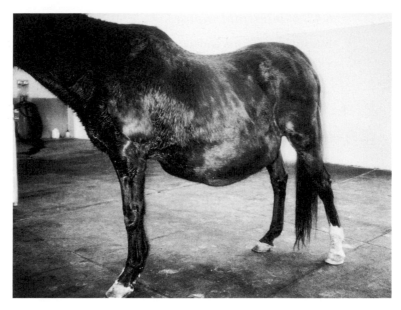

Figure 6.17   Rupture of the pre-pubic tendon may occur in late pregnancy, result-ing in the loss of all abdominal support. The prognosis is not good, death normally results. (Photograph Julie Baumber, © CABI.)

of a heavy pregnancy and this results in a collapse of the abdominal support structures, often resulting in death (Figure 6.17).

6.4.3.2 Prolapse

Prolapse may occur both before and during foaling. Excessive pres-sure in the abdomen forces the vagina, and after parturition, the uterus, to turn inside out and come out through the vulva. If this occurs the vagina and uterus must be wrapped in a clean sheet to support them and keep them as clean as possible, and the veterinary surgeon must be called immediately. The mare will be given a muscle relaxant and the uterus and vagina pushed back and the vulva stitched to keep it in place. Breeding the mare again is not advised.

6.4.3.3 Uterine rupture

Uterine rupture is rare but if it does occur the prognosis for the mare is poor. It may happen before or during parturition and is often the result of a kick or fall in late pregnancy or excessive straining in a mare with a weak uterus.

6.4.3.4 *Intestinal rupture*

Intestinal rupture can occur in late pregnancy or more commonly during parturition and the prognosis for the mare is very poor. It is caused by feeding large infrequent meals which puts excessive strain on the intestines.

6.4.3.5 *Perineal damage and rectal vaginal fissure*

Perineal damage and cuts are common and normally cause no long-term problems. After foaling the vulval area of the mare often appears blue/black with bruising and swelling. Cuts may also be seen but as long as they are only on the surface they should heal well. If there is significant bleeding, e.g. an external haemorrhage, the veterinary surgeon should be called. In extreme cases a rectal vaginal fissure may have been created where the foal's feet have punctured the top of the vagina and passed into the rectum during foaling. This creates a common opening of the vagina and rectum (Figure 6.18). If the fissure

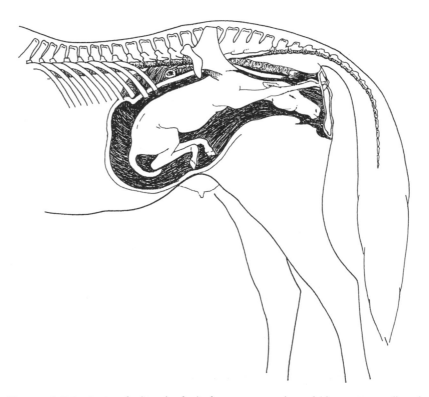

Figure 6.18 During foaling the foal's feet may pass through the vagina wall and up into the rectum, causing a rectal vaginal fissure. © CABI.

is short it may be successfully sewn up but longer ones are difficult to access and the prognosis is very poor.

6.4.3.6 Internal haemorrhage

Internal haemorrhage results from the rupture of the uterine arteries which come under considerable strain at foaling. There is rarely any external sign of bleeding and so the mare may appear well after foaling. However, she will soon show signs of anaemia and low blood pressure, pale mucous membranes, colic, fainting, leading to lack of consciousness and often death. In a few cases the bleeding may stop without any intervention and the mare will slowly recover, however, the majority of cases result in rapid death, although blood transfusions can be attempted. Internal haemorrhage is often the cause if a mare is suddenly found dead after foaling.

6.4.3.7 Retained placenta

In normal circumstances, the placenta gradually reduces in size as the blood flow to it declines; it, therefore, shrinks and separates away from the endometrium. However, especially in mares which have had a difficult foaling, if the placenta is not expelled within the normal 10 hours, the retained placenta will cause infection which, if untreated, will lead to septicaemia, laminitis and death. Veterinary assistance must be sought and treatment usually involves an injection of oxytocin to encourage the uterine muscle to contract along with gentle manipulation, twisting and pulling the placenta to ease its expulsion. Antibiotic pessaries and/or injection must also be given to fight any infection.

6.4.3.8 Post-partum paralysis

Damage can occur to the mare's pelvis and surrounding nerves as a result of frequent standing up and lying down during foaling. This damage makes it difficult for her to stand, and she may appear to be paralysed. She is also in danger of harming herself further and harming the foal, by falling over; so she must be watched carefully. If the pelvis has been dislocated, this can be helped by therapy; if it has been cracked, it will heal in time and nerve damage should also heal slowly of its own accord.

6.4.3.9 Delayed involution

Under normal conditions, within a few hours of foaling, the uterus should have shrunk to one quarter of its fully expanded state. By Day

7 after birth it should be only two to three times the size seen in a barren mare, returning to its normal size by Day 30. In some mares this recovery (*involution*) of the uterus is delayed and causes problems when trying to re-cover the mare (Section 7.6.2, p. 183). Uterine involution can be encouraged by injecting oxytocin and antibiotics combined with gentle exercise.

6.5 CONCLUSION

Correct management of the foaling mare is of utmost importance in ensuring the birth of a healthy foal and the future well-being of the mare. Problems at foaling are rare but inappropriate management, or the failure to call in professional help when required, can have tragic consequences.

Managing the Newborn Foal and the Lactating Mare

7.1 INTRODUCTION

Managing the mare and foal correctly is essential for the long-term well-being of the foal and the rapid recovery of the mare. For the foal, the biggest hurdle to overcome after birth is successfully changing over from a fetus, reliant upon the placenta, to a foal, reliant upon its digestive tract and lungs. This change occurs during what is known as the foal adaptive period.

7.2 FOAL ADAPTIVE PERIOD

Immediately after foaling the foal has to undergo substantial changes in anatomy and function to adapt to its new (extra-uterine) environment. The first four days of life are the most crucial, it is within this period that the majority of adaptation occurs. Many of the adaptive changes can easily be observed by the foaling attendant and failure to meet these changes (*milestones*) within set periods of time can be the first indication of problems (Table 7.1). In a normal birth the foal is born on its side, lying with its hocks still within its mother and the umbilical cord intact (Figure 6.8 (i), p. 147) after this it should rapidly show signs of sitting up (*sternal recumbancy*) (Figure 6.8 (j), p. 147).

7.2.1 Breathing

The foal should take its first breath within thirty seconds of being born. It may take a few sharp intakes of breath as its muzzle first reaches the air during passage through the birth canal, but a rhythm is normally established within one minute of final delivery. These first breaths are stimulated by low blood oxygen (*anoxia*) and high carbon

Table 7.1 A summary of the parameters which should be noted in the first few hours of a foal's life.

Parameter	Average values for the healthy foal (minimum and maximum duration)
Foaling	
Duration of first stage labour	30 minutes (10 minutes–2 days)
Duration of second stage labour	30 minutes (5–60 minutes)
Duration of third stage labour	2 hours (20 minutes–10 hours)
Foal	
Post-partum heart rate	40–80 beats/minute
Resting heart rate (from 24 hours onwards)	80–100 beats/minute
Active heart rate (from 24 hours onwards)	up to 150 beats/minute
Birth to first breath	30–60 secs
Post-partum respiration rate	60–70 breaths/minute
Resting respiration rate (4 hours onwards)	30–40 breaths/minute
Shivering possible	within 3 hours of birth
Birth to breakage of umbilical cord	5–10 minutes
Birth to sitting up (sternal recumbency)	5–15 minutes
Birth to standing	30–90 minutes
Birth to sucking reflex	5–20 minutes
Birth to first suckle	60–120 minutes
Suckle frequency in first few days	1/30–60 minutes
Birth to passing first meconium	0–12 hours
Birth to passing milk dung	48–72 hours
Birth to urination	1–12 hours
Post-partum body temperature	37–37.5°C
Body temperature at 4 hours	38–38.5°C
Weight	7–10% of mare's post-foaling weight 400 kg mare = 28–40 kg foal
Placenta	
Weight	4.5 kg (2.5–6.5 kg depending on mare body weight)

dioxide. Cold shock, from the atmosphere, and tactile stimulus such as rubbing and the mare's licking, also encourage breathing. This initiation of breathing results in an increase in blood oxygen, which encourages muscle movement. The initial breathing rhythm is normally a steady 60–70 breaths/minute but the breaths taken are quite shallow, indicating that breathing is not very efficient. Within a few hours, however, the lungs expand, fluid is expelled and breathing efficiency is increased so the foal begins to breathe more deeply and less rapidly (30–40 breaths/minute at rest).

7.2.2 Heart rate

During the first minute of life the foal's heart rate should be 40–80 beats/minute. This can be measured by placing a hand on the left side of the chest near the heart. The heart rate fluctuates rapidly in the first few hours increasing greatly as the foal struggles to stand and suckle. It may reach up to 150 beats/minute, but a resting heart rate of 80–100 beats/minute should be seen in the first 24 hours.

While in the uterus the placenta acts as the 'lungs' of the foal, being the site of oxygen and carbon dioxide exchange, as well as nutrient uptake. In order to supply the placenta with blood, two by-pass systems are present in the fetal circulatory system; the ductus arteriosus and the foramen ovule (hole in the heart). These ensure that blood is diverted away from the lungs and towards the placenta. As soon as the foal is born these two by-pass systems must close so that blood is sent to the lungs and not the placenta. This happens almost immediately, although many newborn foals may initially suffer from an irregular heartbeat (known as *arrhythmia*), which usually corrects itself within the first few days of life.

Many foals show signs of asphyxia during the second stage of labour, seen as a blue tongue and mucous membranes. This is caused by a reduction in blood flow and, therefore, oxygen, to the head. This is only temporary and within two hours of birth, the mucous membranes should return to their normal pink colour and have a refill time (the time taken to return to a normal pink colour after being pinched) of one to two seconds.

7.2.3 Body temperature

The foal is born with a well-developed temperature control system and from soon after birth can maintain a steady body temperature. At birth the temperature should be 37–37.5°C (100°F), which increases to 38–38.5°C (101°F) within one hour, even in a cold environment. Newborn foals can maintain their body temperature due to their high metabolic rate (three times that of a two-day-old foal); ability to shiver (evident within three hours of birth); muscle activity on standing which generates heat; and the foal's insulating layers of fat together with its hair coat. Hypothermia can occur rapidly in newborn foals, often as a result of infection, dystocia or a very cold environment. Provision of a heat lamp for weak foals in these circumstances can be vital.

7.2.4 Muscle movement

After the stress of birth the foal's first breaths flood its circulatory system with oxygen, this activates the first reflexes and muscle movements. Within five minutes of birth the foal should be sitting up (sternal recumbency position) (Figure 6.8 (j), p. 147). It will respond to pain and begin to show evidence of the reflexes associated with getting

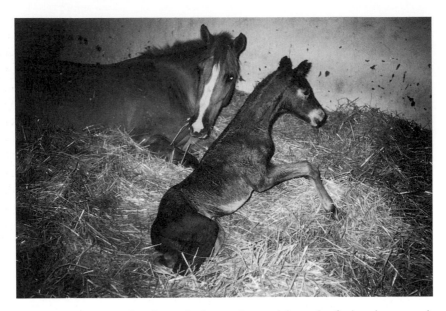

Figure 7.1 Soon after the end of second-stage labour the foal makes several attempts to stand, at this time the umbilical cord breaks. (Photograph Stephen Rufus, © CABI.)

to its feet, raising its head, extending its forelimbs, blinking and possibly a whinny.

7.2.5 Breaking the umbilical cord

It is very important that the cord is allowed to break naturally, as early breakage may result in the loss to the foal of up to 1.5 litres of blood, by preventing drainage of blood from the placenta. In normal conditions the umbilical cord will contract and shrink about 3 cm from the foal's abdomen. In this area the umbilical artery and vein collapse as the blood pressure falls, allowing a clean break and natural sealing, which minimises blood loss and risk of infection. The mare will lean round to lick the foal but may stay lying down for up to 40 minutes, therefore, the cord is usually broken by the movements of the foal as it attempts to stand, usually five to ten minutes after birth. Once the cord has broken it must be dressed with an antiseptic, such as iodine- or chlorohexidine-based preparations.

7.2.6 Standing

The foal makes many unsuccessful attempts to stand as its reflexes and muscle coordination and control develop (Figure 7.1). At this time the

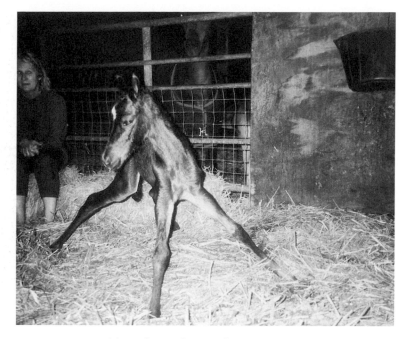

Figure 7.2 Successful standing in the pony foal takes on average 35 minutes compared to up to one hour in the thoroughbred.

foal is at risk of damage from projecting objects such as buckets, hay racks, automatic water feeders etc. Ponies should stand within 35 minutes of birth but thoroughbred-type foals take up to half an hour longer (Figure 7.2). Failure to stand within two hours indicates a problem and veterinary assistance should be sought. This remarkable ability to stand and walk so quickly after birth is the result of the evolution of the horse as a plain-dwelling animal and gives them the ability to flee from predators as soon as possible after birth.

7.2.7 Suckling

Although a foal will suck a finger or teat within five minutes of being born, successful suckling can only occur after it has stood and found the udder. The foal is attracted to dark areas, and the sucking reflex is encouraged by contact with soft, warm surfaces, hence foals are often seen to nuzzle their dam's flanks while searching for the udder (Figure 7.3). The temptation to assist a foal should be resisted as the process of finding the mare's udder can easily be interrupted by human interference. Suckling also represents a major stage in the mare–foal bonding process, as well as providing colostrum. Most mares will help

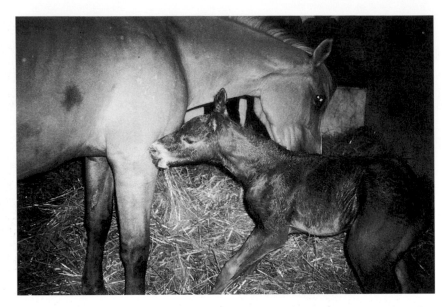

Figure 7.3 Once the foal is standing it is attracted to warm dark areas such as the udder. © CABI.

the foal by gently nudging it and moving her hind leg away from her body to allow the foal easier access. Occasionally, maiden mares appear ticklish and initially object to the foal's attentions, in this case the mare may need to be held to allow the foal to reach the udder.

Ponies should be seen to suckle within sixty minutes, thoroughbreds take on average thirty minutes longer (Figure 7.4). Throughout the first few days of life, the foal will suckle at intervals of fifteen to thirty minutes; later, suckling is less frequent and the amount taken at each session increases. If, during the first few days of life a foal is not seen to suckle for three hours or so, problems should be suspected.

7.2.7.1 Colostrum

The equine placenta is very thick (Section 1.4.3, p. 26) and does not allow the passage of antibodies (immunoglobulins) from the mare to the foal in the uterus. Colostrum is, therefore, vital as the foal's only source of antibodies which provide protection from environmental bacteria. At birth the foal is plunged from the sterile conditions of the uterus into one of bacterial challenge. The foal is perfectly capable of reacting to this challenge, by producing its own antibodies in time, but it is born without any antibodies to act as a 'safety net' until it has produced enough of its own. This 'safety net' is provided by colostrum. However, the antibodies in colostrum can only be absorbed by the

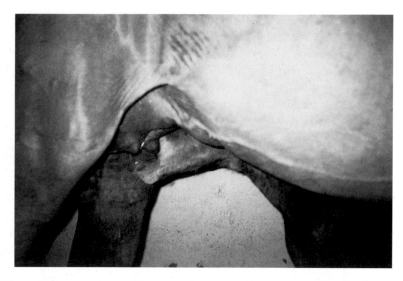

Figure 7.4 In ponies suckling normally occurs within one hour of birth, whereas in thoroughbreds it normally takes one and a half hours. © CABI.

intestine of the foal during the first 24 hours of life, after that they are broken down, like all proteins, into amino acids, before being absorbed. It is essential that newborn foals receive adequate colostrum, at least 500 ml, in the first 24 hours, and ideally within the first 12 hours of life when absorption of antibodies is most efficient. Several blood tests are available to check whether the foal has absorbed enough antibodies and the colostrum itself can be tested to check antibody concentration.

The ability of colostrum to protect the foal can be maximised by making sure that the mare is on the foaling yard four to six weeks before her due date, this allows enough time for her system to raise antibodies to the foaling environment, and for them to be concentrated within the colostrum. It is also good practice to immunise mares (e.g. against influenza and tetanus) in the four to six weeks before parturition so that the antibodies can again pass to the colostrum.

7.2.8 Passage of meconium

During the first twelve hours of life the foal should be seen to pass meconium, its first bowel movement. Meconium is the term given to the greenish-brown bowel secretions which are stored in the colon and caecum of the foal during the last part of pregnancy. Expulsion may occur under stressful conditions during, or immediately prior to, foaling and is seen as meconium staining of the amniotic fluid or the perineum area of the foal and is a sign that the fetus/foal is in distress. In normal conditions meconium is not expelled until after birth and is completely expelled within the first three days, it is followed by the milk dung with its characteristic yellow colour. The passage of the milk dung is a good sign as it indicates that the whole of the foal's gut is functioning correctly. Some studs routinely perform an enema on foals 12–18 hours after birth. However, this is less popular today and considered an unnecessary stress for the newborn foal and is therefore only carried out if meconium retention is suspected.

7.2.9 Urination

The foal should urinate within 12 hours of birth; colts normally urinate earlier than filly foals. Regular urination of small volumes of near colourless urine should be observed in the normal foal.

7.3 POST-FOALING EXAMINATION OF THE FOAL

Within one hour of birth it should be evident whether or not the foal is achieving its milestones (Table 7.1, p. 162), if not, veterinary assistance should be called.

During the post-foaling examination of the foal the following procedures may be carried out:

- Injection of general (broad spectrum) antibiotics (penicillin/ streptomycin)
  - a precautionary action taken by some studs to reduce the chance of infection
- Injection of multivitamins
- Blood testing for:
  - red and white blood cell count
  - isoerythrolysis test: mare–foal compatibility test (Section 7.5.1.5, p. 179)
  - immune status test/antibody uptake test.
- Enema
  - still practised routinely by some, but not advised unless meconium retention is suspected

7.4 EARLY FOAL MANAGEMENT

Management of the lactating mare and foal depends to a certain extent on whether she is to be returned to the stallion or not. If the mare is to foal at stud, her early management and that of the foal, will largely be determined by the general management and practice of the stud. It is, therefore, very important that this is discussed during the selection of a stud.

After the post-foaling examination, the mare and foal should be left in peace with regular, unobtrusive observation. A radiant heat lamp may be used to provide warmth for the foal.

7.4.1 Exercise

For the first three days after birth the eyesight of the foal is not developed enough to safely allow it out of the stable or small foaling paddock. After three days it should be turned out with its dam for an hour or two during the day, providing the weather is good (Figure 7.5). Wet or very cold and windy weather will easily soak the foal and, as both mare and foal will be reluctant to move around in such weather, there is little point in turning them out.

The paddock used should be small, half an acre is ideal. It should have strong, well-constructed fences, ideally, post and three rails with no wire. There should be no protruding objects, old machinery, wire, holes, low branches etc. as these can prove death traps to young foals which are still not sure on their feet.

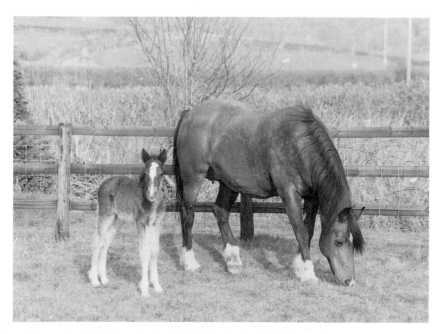

Figure 7.5 After three days a foal's eyesight should have developed enough to allow it to be turned out with its mother.

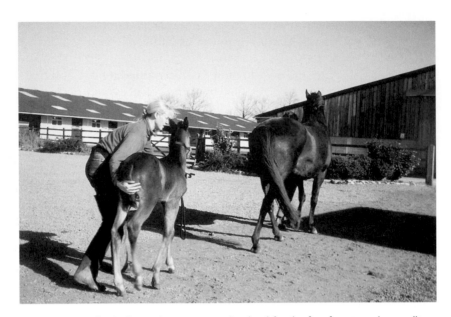

Figure 7.6 The foal may be encouraged to lead for the first few times by cradling it in your arms, one arm behind its hindquarters and the other around its chest. (Photograph Angela Stanfield, © CABI.)

Water should be provided in a bucket. Streams or large water troughs can be dangerous for a very young foal. The paddock should have plenty of good grass, as this will encourage the mare to eat, which is especially important in mares whose appetite has dropped after foaling.

Persuading the foal to leave its stable for the first time can be a challenge, but should be made as stress free as possible. During the first three days the foal should be handled gently, stroked and got used to having arms put around it. If this is carried out then when the big day comes the foal should be used to human contact. The best day to turn a foal out for the first time is a sunny day, but it should not be too hot or flies will be a problem and bright sunlight may discourage the foal from leaving the darker stable. There should be at least two handlers in attendance. The mare should be led ahead slowly by one and the other should cradle the foal in their arms, with one arm behind its hindquarters and the other around its chest, and encourage it to follow its dam (Figure 7.6).

Some foals will follow easily, others prove more difficult. A foal should never be pulled from the head using a halter, as this may damage its neck and head. A soft twisted cloth, bandage or thick rope can be put around its neck initially, to be replaced later with a soft

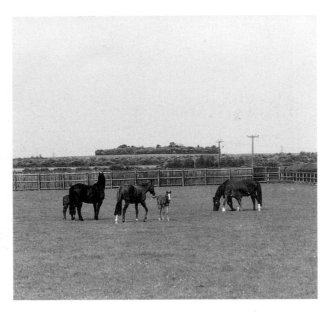

Figure 7.7 Mares and foals are best turned out together in groups to help the foals develop social skills and their ability to interact with other foals and mares.

leather or webbing halter. Leather is preferred as it will eventually break under strain. Head collars can be left on foals and this is convenient for catching them and gives them time to get used to them, however, the collar must be very well fitting to prevent it getting caught on anything including the foal's feet.

As the foal gets older continued turnout is essential to help muscle coordination and development, fitness, gut and heart function, and independence. Ideally, mares and foals should be turned out together in groups to help the foal interact socially (Figure 7.7). Group turnout is an ideal starting point for gradual weaning systems.

7.4.2 Handling

Initial handling in the first few days before turnout should consist of gentle stroking over the whole body and general familiarisation with humans. Some people practice a much more intensive introduction, called imprinting, which is carried out at an hour or so after birth, but after the mare has bonded with the foal by licking it. At this time the foal is introduced to all sorts of stimuli such as, grooming, playing with the ears, clipping, tapping the feet, rectal palpation, loud noises etc., that is everything that the foal might come across in later life. This imprinting habitualises the foal (gets it rapidly used to) to all sorts of

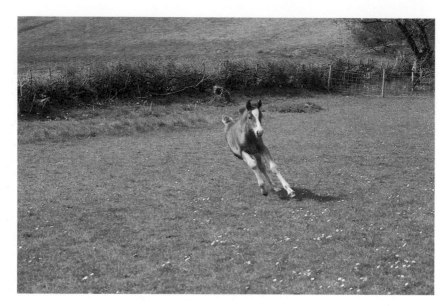

Figure 7.8 Over the first few weeks the foal's circle of play becomes increasingly larger as it gains independence. © CABI.

practices; so that when it comes across them later in life it takes them in its stride. Whether imprinting is used or not a foal must learn early on to accept human attention. Over the first few weeks it should be introduced to grooming, leading, standing still, attention to feet, bathing, tying and, eventually, travelling. These are particularly important if you intend to show the foal.

7.4.3 Behaviour

During the first six weeks of life the foal's behaviour changes as its social interaction develops. Initially the foal's whole world and social experience revolves only around its mother. This includes play, through which it begins to learn how far it can go before being reprimanded and hence what is and is not acceptable. Once the foal has developed more confidence on its feet, after about a week, it will start to explore further away from its mother, but never straying far. Over the next few weeks the circle gets bigger and it spends more time away from its mother, investigating and playing alone (Figure 7.8).

If at this stage the foal has access to other foals it will begin to interact with them and play will gradually include them rather than its mother. By eight weeks it spends up to 50% of its time playing with other foals and only 10% playing around its mother. If, however, the foal has no contact with others it will play with its mother longer and

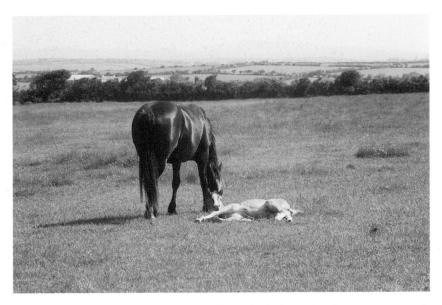

Figure 7.9 In addition to play and suckling, the foal spends a large proportion of its time lying down and resting. © CABI.

may try to play with other older horses or even dogs and other animals regularly in its company. If its mother is particularly possessive, or shy, these characteristics will be picked up by the foal and it will not integrate as well with other foals.

Apart from play, the foal spends a lot of time lying down and resting (Figure 7.9). These are normally short periods of rest, particularly in warm sunlight, between periods of play. The remainder of its time is spent suckling. In the first week these periods of suckling are short and occur every fifteen to thirty minutes. Over time the intervals between sucklings become longer, occurring twenty-five to thirty times/day by week ten, but more milk is taken at each suckle (Figure 7.10).

7.4.4 Nutrition

In theory up until peak lactation (week six to eight) the mare's milk provides the majority of the nutrients required by the developing foal. During this time gradual investigation and eating of the mare's feed provides additional nutrients, but this is not significant until after weeks six to eight. A foal may be seen investigating concentrate feeds as early as three days of age (Figure 7.11). This is to be encouraged, as the mare's milk is naturally short of iron and copper, hence very young foals tend to be anaemic. The foal can get additional copper and iron by picking at the mare's feed. Foals may also be observed nibbling the

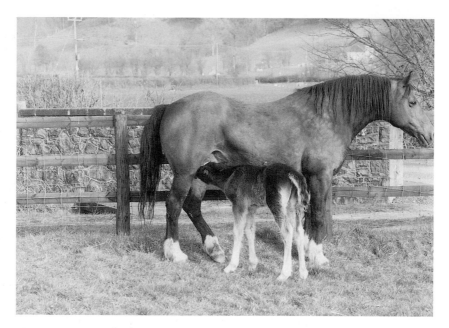

Figure 7.10   As the foal grows it suckles less frequently, but takes more milk at each suckle.

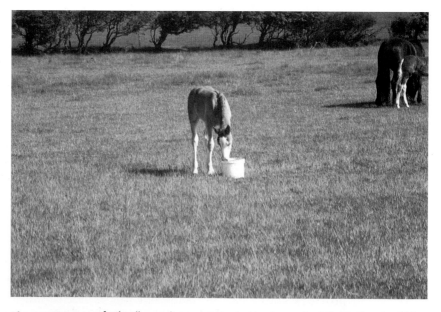

Figure 7.11   A foal will soon be seen investigating its mother's feed. This should be encouraged as it provides the foal with essential copper and iron. © CABI.

mare's dung (known as *coprophagia*). The reason for this is unclear but it may be a way in which the foal obtains minerals or bacteria for its gut. However, this coprophagic behaviour does mean that the foal is at risk of picking up parasites and so the worming of mares with young foals is particularly important (Section 7.4.5, p. 176).

The foal's natural drive to investigate feed is used when introducing it to creep feed (concentrate feed specially formulated for young foals). The amount of creep feed that a foal eats in the first few weeks depends largely on the mare's milk yield. In addition to concentrate creep feed, the foal must be introduced to roughage, grass or hay, since a diet of concentrates and milk alone can cause diarrhoea. Creep feed can be introduced as an optional extra as early as the first week of life, but the foal should never be forced to eat it and the progression from milk to solid food must be gradual. Many commercial creep feeds are available, formulated to give a healthy start in life. These feeds are relatively high in protein (20%) compared to adult diets. Calcium and phosphorus are also of special importance in growing animals as they are essential for healthy bones, cartilage, tendons and joints. Limestone flour can be used to add calcium. In addition to concentrates, foals should have access to fresh, green forage. Hay may be fed, but it must be of a good quality, with no dust, mould, dampness etc. The best option is free access to fresh grass, which provides a continuous ad-lib supply of fresh material. Ideally, the grass should be analysed to make sure that there are no trace mineral deficiencies.

Once the foal starts to pick at its mother's food, care must be taken to ensure that the mare has enough feed to cover her needs, so foals and mares should now be fed individually. Creep feed, due to its high protein content, should also be fed in such a way as to prevent the mare getting access, such as in a creep feeder. By the age of three to four months the foal should be eating around 1 kg of concentrate feed/day about 0.25–1% of its body weight. It is very important to monitor both the foal's intake and condition to avoid obesity, which can lead to excessive strain on young limbs and joints and conditions such as degenerative orthopaedic disease (DOD) (see below).

7.4.4.1 Degenerative orthopaedic disease (DOD)

DOD is the generalised term given to disturbances in skeletal growth and development of foals and youngstock, such as angular limb deformities, contracted tendons etc., incorrect calcification of bone, bone and joint inflammation (osteochondritis dissecans (OC)), vertebral abnormalities and general abnormalities in bone and joint structure and development. There are several causes of DOD including inherited conditions, limb trauma from excessive work on growing limbs, fast growth rates and malnutrition. The last two are the result of incorrect feeding which can have several effects. First, general over-feeding of both energy and protein results in overweight, this leads to excessive strain on young, still growing limbs and joints, causing deformities. Second, incorrect feeding, both too much and too little, of specific nutrients can have specific effects. For example excessive energy appears to have a direct effect on the hormone regulation of bone growth and development. This effect is made worse if animals are fed infrequently, i.e. feeding once a day is more likely to cause DOD than feeding three times a day. Minerals such as calcium and phosphorus are also important, deficiencies of either will cause DOD, in addition the ratio of calcium to phosphorus needs to be correct. If phosphorus levels are relatively high this imbalance will tie up calcium reducing the amount of calcium available for bone growth and, therefore, cause DOD, even if calcium levels in the diet appear correct. Finally copper (Cu) is important for bone growth and development, inadequate levels again leading to DOD.

7.4.5 Parasite control

The worm burden of the young foal will reflect the parasite burden of the mare and the pasture. The mare should undergo regular worming during pregnancy (Section 5.5.3, p. 127) and mares and foals should not be turned out onto pasture which has been grazed by horses within the last twelve months. However, this is often not possible so foals can carry a significant burden of threadworms (*Strongyloides westeri*) and ascarids. Threadworms can cause scouring in two to four-week-old foals, often around foal heat, so foals can be wormed for threadworms from seven days of age (Table 5.4, p. 128). Unfortunately threadworms are fairly resistant to anthelmintics and so relatively high doses are required and there are a limited number of anthelmintics which do work (Table 5.4, p. 128). Ascarids can also be a problem, particularly in foals turned out onto pasture which is used every year for mares and foals. Infested foals lose condition, show slowed growth rate and a dull coat. Treatment with the appropriate anthelmintics (Table 5.4, p. 128) is successful, and by two years of age most horses will have developed resistance to ascarids and so no longer need to be wormed specifically for these.

7.4.6 Vaccinations

Foals can be immunised against tetanus in the first few days of life. However, colostrum, from a suitably immunised mare, is a much more effective way of protecting foals against tetanus and numerous other

Table 7.2   The ages of eruption of equine teeth.

Tooth	Deciduous	Permanent
First incisor	<1 week	2.5 years
Second incisor	4–6 weeks	3.5 years
Third incisor	6–9 months	4.5 years
Canine	–	4–5 years
Wolf tooth	5–6 months	
First cheek tooth	birth–2 weeks	2.5 years
Second cheek tooth	birth–2 weeks	3 years
Third cheek tooth	birth–2 weeks	4 years
Fourth cheek tooth	–	9–12 years
Fifth cheek tooth	–	2 years
Sixth cheek tooth	–	3.5–4 years

diseases. In some countries it may be worth considering immunisation against strangles or rabies depending on how widespread the disease is.

7.4.7 Feet and teeth care

The foal's feet should need little attention in early life unless they have a significant deformity. Nevertheless, picking up the feet, picking out the hooves and grooming the legs should be done regularly. These, along with ensuring a general acquaintance with the blacksmith when the mare's feet are attended to, will make working on the foal's feet later much easier. Regular inspection of the feet will allow examination for injury and damage.

Providing the teeth of the foal erupt as expected and at the correct angle, there is no need to do anything with them in the first six weeks. Most foals are either born with the central incisors or they erupt within eight to nine days, the middle incisors should then erupt at four to six weeks (Table 7.2).

7.5 CONDITIONS OF THE NEWBORN FOAL

Conditions in the newborn (*neonatal*) foal can be divided into non-infective and infective. Whatever the cause, rapid diagnosis of the problem is essential for rapid recovery.

7.5.1 Non-infective conditions

Non-infective conditions normally stem from a problem while the foal was in the uterus.

7.5.1.1 Prematurity

Foals may be born prematurely (early) and so are less able to adapt to life outside the uterus. Prematurity is normally the result of a problem with the mare, fetus or placenta during pregnancy. Diagnosing premature birth is difficult as there is a large range in pregnancy lengths (315–388 days) which result in the birth of a normal foal. It is generally accepted that foals born after a pregnancy of 320 days or less are likely to be premature. Premature foals tend to be underweight, have a characteristic silky coat, have difficulty in breathing, often suffer from colic after suckling and are slow to reach the normal milestones (Section 7.2, p. 161). Providing they are given adequate support premature foals can survive but are often stunted. There are several other conditions which are related to prematurity these include dysmaturity (gestation length appears normal but the foal shows signs of prematurity), intra-uterine growth retardation (gestation length normal but foals are born very thin or stunted).

7.5.1.2 Perinatal asphyxia

Perinatal asphyxia (reduction in oxygen supply to the fetus) can occur during pregnancy, at parturition (if foaling is delayed) or immediately after parturition (when the foal is switching from reliance on the placenta to the lungs), (see also Section 7.5.1.3, p. 178). All foals suffer some asphyxia during parturition, seen as a blue tongue and mucous membranes during birth, but coping mechanisms allow it to be unaffected by such short-term low oxygen levels. Problems occur when low oxygen levels are prolonged, the main organ to be affected is the brain, and hence brain damage is often associated with this condition. The lack of oxygen will also affect other organs and eventually cause death.

7.5.1.3 Neonatal maladjustment syndrome

Neonatal maladjustment syndrome is also known as barkers, wanderers, dummies or convulsives all of which describe very effectively the symptoms in these foals. It is caused by the failure of the foal to adjust to living outside the uterus and in common with perinatal asphyxia results in a lack of oxygen, particularly to the brain. The foal may initially appear normal but may then make a barking-type sound associated with breathing, if it is still lying down it may wave its legs in the air and be unable to stand. Other foals are able to stand but appear uncoordinated, almost blind and are unable to find the teat and suckle. The prognosis for such foals is very poor.

7.5.1.4 Meconium retention

The foal should normally have started to expel meconium within twelve hours of birth and it should all have been expelled within 48–72 hours (Section 7.2.8, p. 167). It is not uncommon for meconium to be retained, such foals can be seen straining with their backs arched and tails up but with no meconium being passed, they may also show signs of colic especially after 24–48 hours. Excessive straining can cause additional problems such as a ruptured bladder (Section 7.5.1.7, p. 180). The condition is normally solved by removing the meconium with a finger placed in the rectum or through use of a simple enema which empties the bowl of meconium and allows the milk dung to be passed. The risk of meconium retention can be reduced by ensuring that the foal has adequate colostrum, which acts as a laxative as well as providing antibodies.

7.5.1.5 Neonatal isoerythrolysis

Neonatal isoerythrolysis is also known as haemolytic anaemia disease or jaundice. During pregnancy some of the blood cells from the fetus may pass across the placenta into the maternal system and if they are incompatible with the mare's blood the mare will raise antibodies against the foal's blood cells. This will not affect the foal during pregnancy but the mare's antibodies, including any against the foal's blood, concentrate in the colostrum. After the foal suckles for the first time these antibodies are absorbed by the intestine, pass into the blood system (Section 7.2.7.1, p. 166) where they then destroy the foal's own red blood cells. This has disastrous consequences, the foal rapidly becoming anaemic, with yellow mucous membranes, red-stained urine and a high pulse and breathing rate, followed by organ failure and death. The condition can be detected by testing the mare's blood for antibodies at two and four weeks before her expected foaling date. If there is evidence of increasing antibodies then the foal must not be allowed to suckle colostrum from its own dam. It must be provided with alternative colostrum from another mare and muzzled for the first 36–48 hours after birth, after which time it can safely suckle its own mother as its digestive tract no longer has the ability to absorb whole antibodies.

7.5.1.6 Circulatory problems

In the fetus there are two bypass mechanisms (the foramen ovule (hole in the heart) and the ductus arteriosus) which ensure that blood is passed to the placenta rather than the lungs. Immediately after birth these two bypasses must close to ensure that the fetal circulatory system switches to a foal circulatory system sending blood to the lungs. Occasionally the closure of the two bypasses does not occur immediately and the foal appears listless and is slow to achieve its milestones. However, the prognosis is good and the condition often cures itself within a few days.

7.5.1.7 Ruptured bladder

Occasionally so much pressure builds up in the foal's abdomen either during birth or as a result of constant straining from retained meconium, that the bladder ruptures. Such foals will show signs of colic, a distended abdomen and not be seen to pass urine. This is a serious condition but as long as it is diagnosed quickly surgery can be effective.

7.5.1.8 Pervious urachus

The urachus is a tube which passes from the bladder of the fetus along the umbilical cord and empties into the allantoic sac. At birth it normally seals and urine is then stored in the bladder, occasionally it fails to close and urine leaks from the umbilical region. This can cause infection, inflammation and soreness. Surgery is required and is very effective.

7.5.1.9 Umbilical hernia

An umbilical hernia, a swelling in the naval region of the foal, is caused by a weakness in the abdominal wall forming a bulge in the skin. In the worst cases a section of intestine may become trapped in this opening and lie within the pocket of skin, there is the risk that the intestine may become trapped and a blockage caused in the intestine followed by eventual 'death' of part of the gut and subsequently the foal. However, surgery is very successful in such cases and less severe cases often eventually heal without intervention.

7.5.1.10 Contracted/extended tendons

Contracted tendons are not uncommon in foals and are evident to varying degrees. The condition arises when the tendons, most commonly in the forelegs, are too short for the cannon bone causing the foal's foot to be permanently bent backwards. In most cases the foal is born with the condition but occasionally it can occur after birth. The prognosis for very severe cases is poor and such foals have to be destroyed, however, many cases are not as severe and can be successfully treated by exercise, massage, strapping and therapy. Extended tendons are the opposite to contracted tendons: tendons are too long and as a result the fetlock joint touches the ground. This condition is not as severe as contracted tendons and invariably cures itself with time.

7.5.2 Infective conditions

Infections can stem from a problem both in the uterus and during early life. It may be the only problem affecting a foal or is often seen in foals that already have non-infective problems (Section 7.5.1, p. 177). The cause of the infection is normally a bacterium or virus (Table 7.3) which has entered the mare's reproductive tract during pregnancy, or has entered the foal soon after birth through the respiratory or gastrointestinal system, or the umbilical cord. Rapid treatment is successful particularly if the specific bacteria involved can be identified and a targeted antibiotic used. Broad spectrum antibiotics are commonly used as a preventive measure, but this overuse leads to bacterial resistance to antibiotics.

7.6 MANAGEMENT OF THE MARE

Immediately after foaling the mare should be left in peace to bond with her foal. She should have a good supply of hay or fresh grass and clean water. After an hour or so she may be given a small nutritious feed. She should then be left and observed from a distance. Apart from a post-foaling examination (Section 7.6.2, p. 183) and any handling of the foal the mare should just be monitored carefully in the first few weeks to make sure that she has not suffered any long-term detrimental effects of pregnancy.

7.6.1 Milk production

About 72 hours after foaling the mammary gland starts to produce milk rather than colostrum (Section 1.5, p. 30). During the start of lactation it is important that the mare looks healthy and is fit in herself, as any infections or disease will easily pass to the foal. The general well-being of the foal should also be used as an indication of milk production. If the mare is not producing enough milk the foal will appear 'tucked up', the mare's teats may be sore from continual

Table 7.3 Some common infective conditions of the young foal adapted from Rossdale, P. and Ricketts S.W., *Equine Stud Farm Medicine* (1980). Ballière and Tindall, Eastbourne, UK.

Condition	Synonyms	Characteristics	Cause
Generalised infections	Diarrhoea/ Scours Pleurisy Pneumonia Peritonitis	Fever to 39.5°C (102°F) and persisting Diarrhoea Increased respiratory rate with rales Dehydration, retraction of eyeballs	*Escherichia coli* *Streptococcus* spp.
Hepatitis	Virus abortion Rhinopneumonitis	Convulsions Lethargy Mild jaundice	*Equid herpesvirus-1* *Cytomegalovirus*
Nephritis	Viscosum Shigellosis Sleepy foal disease Sleeper	Initial fever to 102°F (39.5°C) becoming subnormal ↓ suck strength Diarrhoea, mild colic Convulsions Uraemia: protein/blood cells in urine	*Actinobacillus equuli* (BVE)
'Meningitis'	Convulsions	Fever to 39.5°C (102°F) and persisting Convulsions	*Streptococcus* spp. *Escherichia coli* *Actinobacillus equuli*
Encephalitis		Gross disturbances in behaviour	General infection/ inflammation of the brain = fluid accumulation = ↑ pressure = ↑ head size
Infective arthritis	Joint ill Navel ill	Fever to 39.5°C (102°F) and persisting Lameness	*Streptococcus* spp. *Salmonella typhimurium*
Tenosynovitis		Painful swelling around joints	*Staphylococcus* spp. *Escherichia coli*

unsuccessful suckling and she may begin to object to the foal. Low milk yields may be due to a physical inability, poor feeding or body condition, or mastitis.

Mastitis, an infection of the mammary gland, is rare but may occur both after foaling and also at weaning. The mastitic udder is hot, swollen and painful with fluid collecting along the abdomen and between the hind legs. The milk tends to be thick and clotted and should not be fed to foals. Treatment is similar to that in cows, by the administration of antibiotics directly into the mammary gland through the streak canal, with treatment repeated for several days.

7.6.2 Post-foaling examination of the mare and mating on the foal heat

An internal examination of the mare is often carried out within three days of foaling to identify any problems and check uterine involution (recovery) (Section 6.4.3.9, p. 159). Any problems can then be treated in time for either, covering at the foal heat (first oestrus after foaling), or the second oestrus. The mare may now be given a Caslick's (Section 1.2.2, p. 3) either to replace clips put in the vulva immediately after foaling or if her vulva is damaged.

In many studs, especially thoroughbred studs, there is pressure to get one foal per mare per year, with each foal born as early in the season as possible (Section 2.2.1.2.1, p. 43) which means that the mare needs to be re-covered as soon as possible after foaling. Most mares show foal heat 4–10 days after foaling. However, uterine involution has a significant effect on conception rates and so a rapid recovery is essential if the uterus is to accept a new pregnancy so soon. Uterine involution involves the return of the uterus to its pre-pregnancy size and recovery of the uterine endometrium. Normally by seven days the uterus has reduced to two or three times its non-pregnant size and by Day 30 should be back to normal. Endometrium recovery is slower, but again should be complete by Day 30. Full uterine involution must have occurred if the best conception rates are to be achieved. Foal heat at 4–10 days after foaling does not, therefore, allow enough time for the uterus to recover fully, so conception rates are normally poor. Ideally, mares should not be covered until at least 10 days after foaling, whether that be on her foal heat or the second oestrus after foaling. This can be achieved by: delaying the foal heat by treating the mare with progesterone for 10 days or so after foaling; or waiting until the second oestrus to cover the mare.

7.6.3 Exercise

Mares and foals should be turned out about three days after foaling (Section 7.4.1, p. 169). Exercise is important in helping the uterus to recover especially in the first few days after foaling and is associated with better conception rates. Feral ponies have good conception rates at foal heat; this is possibly because they are free to exercise at will, compared to domesticated mares which are housed for much of the time.

7.6.4 Nutrition

Nutrition is particularly important in the lactating mare as she has higher requirements than any other horse, even one in heavy work. As parturition approaches, her demand for nutrition increases to satisfy the needs of the growing fetus (Section 5.5.2, p. 121). After parturition the mare continues to provide all the nutrients for the foal, but now these must reach the foal via milk and in addition the foal now requires higher levels of nutrients. Supplying nutrients via milk is less efficient than via the placenta and so the mare's requirements increase rapidly (Tables 5.2, p. 124 and 5.3, p. 126). At peak lactation a mare may produce up to 3% of her body weight as milk (8–12 litres/day for a pony or 10–18 litres/day for thoroughbreds). As with the pregnant mare, protein and energy are important, under-feeding of either will cause milk production to drop and result in an ill thrifty foal.

In general the nutrient requirements of the mare are determined by her level of milk production and the length of her lactation, i.e. the shape of the lactation curve (Section 1.5.2, p. 33 and Figure 1.35, p. 34). The lactation curve is in turn determined by the demands of the foal, i.e. its size, appetite, activity, whether creep feed is being fed and when weaning occurs. In addition there is considerable variation between mares, some mares do their foals very well by producing a lot of milk and so have higher nutritional demands. Some mares may also have been put back in foal during this period; however, due to the low additional nutrient requirements of early pregnancy (Section 5.5.2, p. 121) and the overwhelming extra requirements for lactation, both barren lactating mares and pregnant lactating mares can be fed the same ration. It is very difficult, therefore, to state exactly what the nutrient requirements for the lactating mare are. However, in general, lactation can be divided into two periods, the period up to and just after peak lactation (usually two to three months after parturition) when milk production and hence the mare's requirements are at their greatest (discussed here), and the period after peak lactation until weaning (usually at six months in managed horses) when the foal is increasingly less reliant on milk and hence milk production and the mare's nutrient requirements are falling (Section 8.3.1, p. 192).

During the first part of lactation nutrient requirements in the mare are at their highest, the demand for energy in particular increases by up to 100% when compared to maintenance requirement. During the first three months of lactation a 500 kg mare needs 28.3 MCal/day compared to 16.4 MCal/day for maintenance or 19.7 MCal/day in the last month of pregnancy (Table 5.2, p. 124). Protein requirements also increase significantly and are often underestimated causing deficiency in the diets of many lactating mares. Requirements increase to 1427 g CP (crude protein)/day for a 500 kg mare in the first three months of lactation compared to 656 g CP/day for maintenance and 866 g CP/day in the last month of pregnancy (Table 5.2, p. 124). In order to meet these demands the mare will need to be fed a feed containing an average of 2.6 MCal/kg and with a protein content of 13.2% (Table 5.3, p. 126). This can rarely be achieved by forage alone, even very good forage and so concentrates invariably need to be fed. Calcium and phosphorus, due to their link with foal bone and tendon growth (Section 7.4.4.1, p. 175) particularly are important in the lactating mare's diet. Again her requirements significantly increase to 56 g/day for calcium and 36 g/day for phosphorus, from late pregnancy requirements of 37 g/day for calcium and 28 g/day for phosphorus (Table 5.2, p. 124) and are likely only to be satisfied by feeding concentrate feeds. Vitamins A and D are necessary to the foal and are obtained via milk and so are important components of the early lactating mare's diet. Vitamin A is found in fresh green forage and vitamin D from exposure to sunlight, so turning mares and foals out onto fresh pasture in springtime is a good way of ensuring the presence of these vitamins. Even so many studs routinely provide their mares with supplements which can also include calcium and phosphorus. Lastly, but by no means least, free access to clean fresh water at all times is essential, as 90% of milk is in fact water.

As with all feeding a mare may lose or gain condition during lactation despite being fed an apparently ideal ration. Hence her body condition should always be monitored and her feed adjusted accordingly to ensure that she remains fit not fat with a body condition score of 3 (Section 3.4, p. 66).

7.6.5 Parasite control

As with all adult horses the lactating mare with a young foal at foot is susceptible to large and small strongyles, bots, tapeworm, lungworm and pinworm. However, foals are particularly susceptible to ascarids and threadworms (Section 7.4.5, p. 176) and so wormers which also act against these are advised, especially if a problem is suspected (Table 5.4, p. 128). The mare's worming should also fit in with the worming of other stock on the stud and a system of clean grazing and dung removal practised (Section 5.5.3, p. 127).

7.6.6 Vaccination

No specific vaccination of mares is required during early lactation, providing the mare has been adequately vaccinated in late pregnancy.

7.6.7 Teeth and feet care

Teeth and feet care continue to be important and their care should be continued as normal.

7.7 CONCLUSION

Correct management of the young foal and lactating mare will ensure that the foal has the best start in life and that the mare is in a fit condition to be successfully re-covered and carry another pregnancy.

Managing the Older Foal and Weaning

8.1 INTRODUCTION

The life of the older foal is dominated by increasing independence from its mother both physically (no longer relying on mare's milk) and psychologically (interacting with other foals and horses rather than just its mother).

8.2 MANAGEMENT OF THE OLDER FOAL

From six weeks of age onwards the foal becomes increasingly independent of its mother, and management of the foal at this stage must reflect this.

8.2.1 Exercise

Turnout is essential to help muscle coordination and development, fitness, digestive and circulatory system function, and independence. It is best if mares and foals are turned out together in groups. This will help the foal's social awareness and appreciation of hierarchy, and is also an ideal starting point for gradual weaning systems.

8.2.2 Handling

Handling of the foal should continue to develop and reinforce the firm basis laid down in early life. Halter breaking should be well established (Figure 8.1). Leading lessons should develop this and well before weaning the foal should be happy to be led without resistance both behind and away from its mother. This can only be achieved by continuous and patient training, using short, frequent lessons

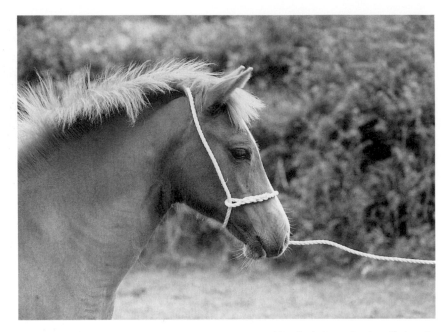

Figure 8.1 Halter breaking is important in the older foal if it is be handled with safety. © CABI.

(Figure 8.2). The foal should also be accustomed to travelling in company and then alone.

8.2.3 Behaviour

The older foal continues to develop its independence, spending time away from its mother, playing and interacting with other foals. This is invaluable in developing social awareness and in preparation for survival on its own with other horses.

8.2.4 Nutrition

From about two to three months of age onwards forage and hard feed (often creep feed) become an increasingly important component of the foal's diet. From this stage onwards the mare's milk quality declines, encouraging the foal to seek nutrients elsewhere. The quality of creep feed fed must be carefully assessed to ensure that it provides all the nutrients required for optimum growth and development. It must be remembered that optimum growth is required not maximum growth.

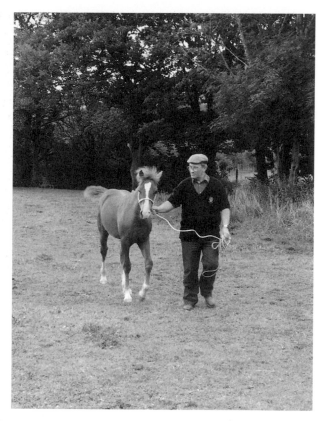

Figure 8.2 The foal should learn to lead without resistance from an early age. (Photograph Penpontbren Welsh Cob Stud, © CABI.)

The period of fastest growth is three to six months when, as a rough guide, a foal destined to make 15–16 hh (150–160 cm), 400–500 kg in weight may gain 1 kg to 2 kg/day. Growth rate then slows between six and twelve months to 0.5 kg/day. By one year of age the foal should not weigh more than 80% ideally (60–70%) of its expected mature weight (320–400 kg) and will have reached around 90% of its mature height. From twelve months of age growth rate slows further and so weight is gained more slowly until mature size is achieved around four to five years of age. The foal does not only increase in weight and size but there is a variation in which structures grow when. The first structures to grow and mature are the bones, followed by muscle and finally fat until growth is complete at mature size. The diet must, therefore, reflect these changing growth patterns, so although all components of the diet are essential (protein, energy and minerals) there are times when certain nutrients are particularly important, for example in the youngest animals (the first three months) nutrients for bone growth are of prime importance (calcium and phosphorus), followed in slightly older animals (around six months) with a particular requirement for nutrients for muscle growth (protein), followed finally by a higher requirement for nutrients for fat deposition (carbohydrates or energy in the diet).

Careful rationing and a matching of feed to requirements is necessary in order to maintain development and also to avoid excessive weight gain which puts strain on muscles, tendons, joints, the circulatory system etc. This is especially important at this stage, while these structures are still developing, as undue stress can cause permanent deformity. As with younger foals the need for quality protein, calcium and phosphorus is high. Creep feeds (Section 7.4.4, p. 173) normally contain 20% protein, 2.9 Mcal/kg energy, 0.8% calcium and 0.6% phosphorus. The quality of protein as well as the quantity is particularly important in growing foals, as protein, together with calcium and phosphorus is essential for bone growth and development.

The adequate supply of essential amino acids such as lysine (those which the body cannot make itself) is extremely important to youngstock. Even if the total protein content of the diet is correct, the horse may still suffer from protein deficiency due to the lack of an essential amino acid. Lysine is often deficient in youngster's diets. At three months the foal requires 15 g lysine/day (Table 5.2, p. 124), though fresh green forage may have adequate levels of lysine, they are often very variable and, therefore, concentrate feeds with a high lysine content 0.6–0.7% should be fed. As the foal gets older its total intake of forage and concentrates increases and by four months of age, even though its total daily requirements will still be increasing, the concentration of nutrients within the whole diet can be reduced. Concentrate feeds for older foals normally have a lower protein concentration (16%) than creep feeds even though the total protein requirement for a moderately growing youngster at six months (750 g/day) is greater than at four months (720 g/day) (Table 5.2, p. 124).

At two months of age 0.5 kg of creep feed per day is adequate, by three months foals should be consuming 0.3–0.5 kg/100 kg bodyweight/day (about 1 kg/day). It is important that the mare cannot eat the creep feed as this may discourage the foal from eating and in addition creep feed has a higher protein concentration (20%) than the mare requires (11%). Specially designed creep feeders are available which allow the foal to feed undisturbed by the mare. The amount of feed per foal should be monitored and if foals are run out in a group it is best if possible for them to be fed individually. This may prove difficult but will ensure that each foal is fed according to its need and adjusted to its weight gain. Free access to creep feed allows greedy foals to gorge themselves at the expense of smaller less dominant indi-

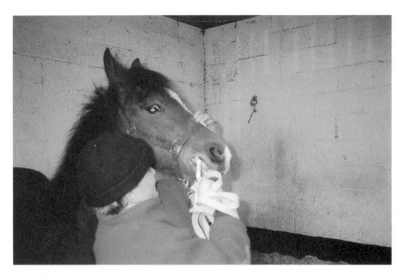

Figure 8.3   Regular worming should be established by two months of age and continue as a routine for the rest of the foal's life. © CABI.

viduals. Free access to fresh grass or forage is essential and access to a mineral supplement is good practice.

8.2.5 Parasite control

Older foals are susceptible to all the worms which infest adult horses: large and small strongyles, bots, tapeworm, lungworm and pinworm (Section 5.5.3, p. 127) but they will not have yet developed resistance to ascarids. Worming older foals should, therefore, not only follow the same principles used when worming adult animals (Section 5.5.3, p. 127) but should also include wormers active against ascarids (Table 5.4, p. 128). A regular worming regime should be established from three months of age and from then on all youngsters should be wormed with other animals on the stud as part of a regular worming programme and a clean grazing policy followed (Figure 8.3).

8.2.6 Vaccination

Until four to five months of age the best protection against the more common diseases, such as tetanus and influenza, is provided by colostrum (Section 7.2.7.1, p. 166). After this, vaccination should be started. Immunisation against strangles or rabies may be considered in the older foal depending on disease prevalence.

8.2.7 Teeth and feet care

Foot problems can be identified and possible correction considered within the foal's first year of life. In addition to regular trimming and handling, this can ensure that minor faults and problems can be identified before training begins. Over zealous care of a young foal's feet, should be avoided as it can make existing problems worse. Indeed, many problems will correct themselves given time. Corrective trimming should only be done by a trained and experienced farrier or veterinary surgeon. Deformities, such as an incorrect hoof, pastern angle toes out or in, excessively long toes or club foot can all be helped by corrective trimming.

By six weeks the foal's first and second incisors should have erupted. The wolf teeth then follow at five to six months, followed by the third deciduous incisors at six to nine months (Table 7.2, p. 177). Attention to teeth beyond familiarisation with opening the mouth to allow the teeth to be viewed should not be required at this stage.

8.3 MANAGEMENT OF THE LACTATING MARE WITH AN OLDER FOAL

From about two to three months after parturition lactation yield decreases, along with the foal's reliance upon its dam for food and psychological support. This should be reflected in the management of the mare.

8.3.1 Nutrition

From two to three months of age onwards the foal demands increasingly less milk as it becomes more reliant upon solid feeds, hence milk yield declines and there is a reduction in the mare's requirement for nutrients. At this stage some mares may also be up to three months pregnant with next year's foal. However, as in the case of the early lactating mare (Section 7.6.4, p. 184) the limited increased demand for pregnancy at this stage (Section 5.5.2, p. 121) and the overwhelming extra requirements for lactation mean that barren lactating mares and pregnant lactating mares can be rationed in the same way. So whether she is pregnant or not the decreasing demand for milk from the foal must be reflected in the mare's feed. In particular the energy concentration of the diet can be reduced, for example for a 500 kg mare from 2.6 MCal/kg to 2.45 MCal/kg as the requirements drop from 28.3 MCal/day to 24.3 MCal/day (Table 5.2, p. 124). Similarly protein concentrations can be reduced from 13.2% to 11% as the mare's daily requirements drop from 1427 g to 1048 g, calcium and phosphorus requirements also decline (Table 5.2, p. 124). The levels of all these nutrients can be dropped still further as weaning approaches and can at this stage largely be met by good quality forage, and fresh pasture, with little need for concentrate feeds.

Finally water must not be forgotten: the mare's requirement for free access to fresh clean water remains high throughout lactation.

As with all feeding a mare's body condition should also be monitored for excessive loss or gain, which may occur despite being fed an apparently ideal ration. Her feed must then be adjusted to ensure that she remains fit not fat, with a body condition score of 3 (Section 3.4, p. 66).

8.3.2 Exercise

Exercise at this stage is essential in order to build up the mare's fitness after parturition. The mare and the foal should be turned out for as long as is possible, ideally day and night. If the weather is too hot they may be brought in during the day to avoid the flies and be turned out at night.

8.3.3 Vaccination, parasite control, teeth and feet care

Worming regime, vaccination programmes, attention to teeth and feet should not be neglected and maintained as normal (Sections 5.5.3, p. 127, 5.5.4, p. 129 and 5.5.5, p. 130), to ensure that the mare remains in optimum condition.

8.4 WEANING

Correct weaning and youngstock management is crucial to the foal's long-term health, physical growth and development, psychological development and social interaction with other horses and humans. Weaning is essential to allow the mare's udder to recover in time for the next foal. In natural conditions the foal would be weaned at nine to ten months of age, giving the mare at least one month to recover before the birth of the new foal. By nine months the foal will be eating mainly solid food with minimum milk intake. This dry period, after weaning and before the new lactation, allows the mare's system to recover, concentrate on supporting the foal she is now pregnant with and rebuild body reserves.

8.4.1 The timing of weaning

In the wild, the six-month-old foal derives most of its nutrients from grass and herbage. It is therefore quite possible, with careful management and the provision of a creep feed, to wean healthy foals at six months. This is practiced by most studs providing the foal is in good physical condition and is eating adequate amounts of concentrates. The time of weaning will also depend upon the mare's behaviour, month of foaling and the dependence of the foal upon the mare. Early weaning, as early as four months of age, may be considered if the mare is losing condition, ill or producing little milk. Providing the weaning is well planned, the foal is well prepared, introduced to solids soon enough and in good physical condition, neither mare or foal should suffer.

Weaning is a potentially very stressful process for the foal, both physically and psychologically. It will be separated from its dam, milk will be excluded from its diet, it may be introduced to unfamiliar horses and there will be more handling and contact with humans. However, with careful management these stresses can be reduced. Physical stress can be minimised by ensuring that the foal is eating enough solid food and that the switch from milk is gradual (Figure 8.4). Sudden changes in diet at all ages can cause digestive upsets and in foals can lead to a reduction in growth and development. For this reason foals can be fed milk pellets for a while after weaning.

It is important that the foal is in good health prior to weaning. Any animals showing signs of illness, such as runny nose, coughing, listlessness, starry coat, diarrhoea etc. must not be weaned until their condition improves. Young animals are particularly susceptible to seemingly minor problems which slow their development, and may cause permanent damage. If in doubt, it is always advisable to call a veterinary surgeon.

Psychological stress is also a potential problem but can be reduced by introducing the foal to his post-weaning companions and regular handling before separation from his mother.

8.4.2 Methods of weaning

There are four main types of weaning: sudden or abrupt; gradual; interval or paddock; and weaning in pairs. The method used is dictated by the facilities available, the numbers of foals and youngstock and also by personal preference. Traditionally, foals were weaned suddenly, although recently the other methods, which are based upon a more gradual removal of the mare or the introduction of other companions, have been recommended.

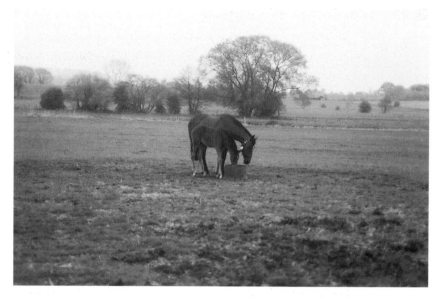

Figure 8.4 Intake of solid food must be adequate prior to weaning. This will minimise the upset to the digestive system of the foal as a result of the change from a liquid-milk based to solid concentrate and forage-based diet.

8.4.2.1 Sudden or abrupt weaning

Sudden or abrupt weaning involves the abrupt separation of the mare and foal. For this system of weaning a safe and secure stable is required, free from projections and water buckets either fixed to the wall or left unattended. Hay should be fed in a rack off the ground, a hay net is not advised as the foal may strangle itself; hay on the floor is better but can be wasted. The bed should be deep, ideally made of straw, providing good protection if the foal launches around the box. The stable door should be secure with an upper grill or metal mesh door as well as a solid upper door (Figure 8.5).

At weaning the mare is quickly taken out of the stable leaving the foal behind. The foal should by now be used to handling and can be held in the stable while the mare is removed. She must be kept moving even though she is likely to be very reluctant, the quicker she is removed and with the least fuss the better. As soon as she is out of the stable both solid doors top and bottom should be shut and the stable light left on. The foal should be relatively safe under these conditions for a short while until the mare has been attended to.

The mare should be taken to a field out of earshot of the foal, with limited grass cover. The field should be secure with safe boundaries. Some mares are very disturbed for the first few hours and career

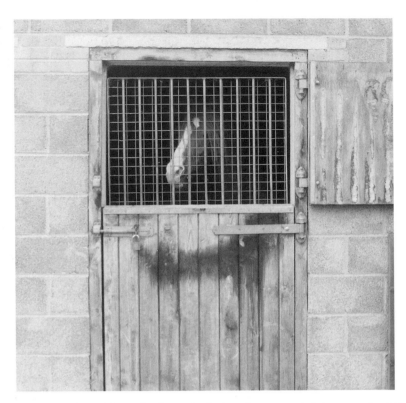

Figure 8.5 The stable used to leave the foal in after removal of the mare should be very secure and have an upper grill or mesh as well as a solid upper door. © CABI.

around wildly, others appear to be relieved. The mare should be watched until she has settled down and the foal then checked. The foal should be given water as it will no doubt have worked itself into a good 'lather'. Hay should be fed *ad libitum* along with a small concentrate feed as soon as it has calmed down. It should remain in the box for the first few days to allow it to get used to life alone. A large stable is, therefore, a good idea. For these first few days the upper mesh door should be closed at all times to prevent the foal from attempting to jump out and yet still provide ventilation. Foals are notoriously unaware of danger and will launch themselves at obstacles that an adult horse would not dream of attempting. They are, therefore, very prone to damage and extra care should be taken to avoid potential hazards: prevention is better than cure. The foal should be handled and mucked out regularly.

These first few days are very stressful for the foal and it is susceptible to physical damage and disease, and this is one of the main disadvantages of this system. After a few days, providing the foal is calm, it may be turned out for short periods in a small, secure paddock with a companion. The length of turnout can be increased gradually until the foal is out all day and night, though in many systems foals are still brought in at night through until the following spring since weaning occurs during late summer or autumn.

During this time the mare should not be neglected. Her udder may start to show signs of tenderness and discomfort due to the increase in milk pressure. A small amount of milk can be milked out of the udder each day for the first few days in order to reduce the pressure and hence the chance of mastitis. The amount of milk removed daily should only be small and should be gradually reduced over five days. The removal of too much milk only serves to prolong the problem. If milk build-up within the udder leads to excessive pressure, infection and mastitis can result. Mastitis in mares is relatively rare but if it occurs it can prove fatal if not treated appropriately. Antibiotic treatment is usually successful, although there is always the danger of the infected part of the udder being lost.

8.4.2.2 Gradual weaning

Gradual weaning is an increasingly popular method of weaning as it attempts to reduce the stresses of sudden weaning. It can be practised in yards with single mares or groups (Figure 8.6). If two stables are to be used for the mare and foal they must, as with abrupt weaning, be safe and secure and ideally have an interconnecting barred window. More commonly, adjacent paddocks are used, these again need to be well fenced and secure, preferably one more lush for the foal, as its requirements will be greatest and eating will provide a distraction. Initially, the mare and foal are turned into the separate paddocks or stables for a short period of time, half an hour or so. Over the next couple of weeks this time of separation increases until they are turned out separately all the time. The closeness of the foal to the mare allows physical contact and emotional security but does not allow suckling. Independence and a reduction in milk intake are developed over time and so the stress of abrupt complete separation is much reduced. An added advantage of this system is that as the time of separation is gradually increased mastitis is not a problem.

8.4.2.3 Paddock or interval weaning

Paddock weaning requires careful planning and is not possible with single foals or with foals of vastly differing ages. In an ideal situation foals should be born in batches within two weeks of one another and

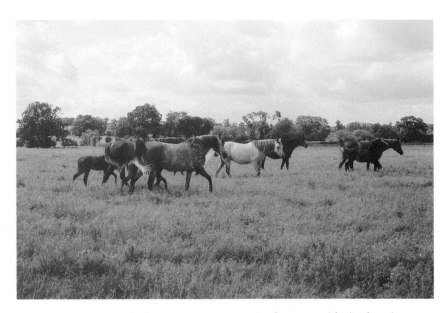

Figure 8.6 In a gradual weaning system groups of mares and foals of similar ages are run together in preparation for the gradual removal of the mares at weaning. © CABI.

brought up together. This allows them to become accustomed to each other and a hierarchy developed while their mothers are still present to reduce any aggression. Near the time of weaning all foals should be checked for physical condition and adequate solid food intake. In an ideal system on large studs there will also be other batches of younger foals born later and following behind so any foals not ready for weaning in one batch can be transferred to the next one, giving them an extra two more weeks or so to become prepared.

Once all the foals are ready for weaning, the most dominant mare or the dam with the most independent foal is removed on one day, followed by the next most dominant the next day etc. until all have been removed. A placid dry mare may then be introduced to the group as a companion. The mares must be taken well away from the foals and out of earshot. The foal which has lost his mother soon forgets due to the solace and security of his fellow foals and the other mares. Mares should again be watched for mastitis.

8.4.2.4 Weaning in pairs

A final alternative, though not widely used, is paired weaning. Based upon the sudden weaning system, foals are weaned abruptly in pairs

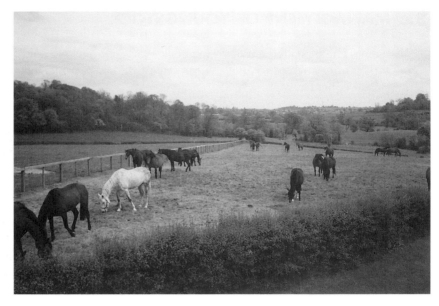

Figure 8.7 After weaning, mares can be turned out into a paddock with limited grass cover to help dry up their milk production.

rather than singles, two foals being left in a stable together. However, this system does require the two foals to be 'weaned' from each other at a later stage, which may be as stressful as initial sudden weaning alone would have been.

8.5 CARE OF THE MARE AFTER WEANING

The mare's udder should be watched for evidence of tenderness as a result of milk accumulation. In order to minimise this she should be turned out into a paddock with limited grass cover and not be provided with any concentrate feed (Figure 8.7). This limits her nutritional intake and forces her to exercise in order to obtain what grass she eats. Exercise helps to relieve pressure in the udder and uses nutrients which would otherwise have gone towards milk production. Her paddock should be secure and free from hazards as some mares may initially be agitated at the loss of the foal. The mare usually recovers quicker from the separation than the foal and, in some cases, may even seem relieved to be free of the extra burden.

8.6 MANAGEMENT OF YOUNGSTOCK

The management of youngstock is a vast topic and so this section will only attempt to give a summary of the main principles and points to consider.

8.6.1 Exercise

As previously discussed, exercise and social interaction with other horses is essential for a youngster's physical and psychological development. Youngsters should be reared at pasture and this practice is becoming increasingly widespread (Figure 8.8). Such animals can exercise at will, reducing the strain on growing bones, allowing muscles and tendons to develop and grow in strength and size. Social interaction with other horses develops a respect for fellows and reduces boredom and stops the development of the bad habits of confinement. Bad weather and lack of available land are often the reason for restricted turnout. Conditions such as heavy rain, snowfall and driving wind or very hot weather may justify youngsters being brought inside. The only major disadvantage of pasture-kept youngsters is the difficulty in making sure that all have an adequate intake of concentrates. Most studs feed a standard ration to all pasture-kept

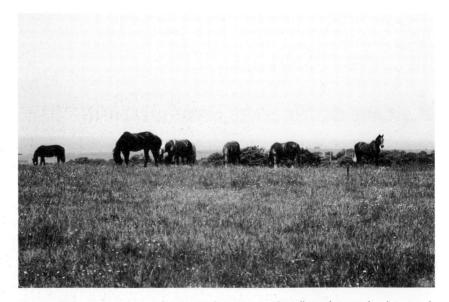

Figure 8.8   Youngsters are best reared at pasture. This allows them to develop social interaction and respect for others, as well as providing exercise, to the advantage of bone, muscle and tendon development. © CABI.

youngsters together and any individuals which appear to be in under- or over-condition are fed separately.

8.6.2 Housing

The nutritional requirements of any youngster are partly determined by its environment and housing. The higher the maintenance requirement of the horse, the higher its nutrition requirements. Nutrition required for maintenance increases if the weather is bad, i.e. wind, rain, cold etc., so the overall ration must be increased to compensate. If this is not done then the growth and development of the horse will be adversely affected. In order to minimise maintenance requirements and hence feed costs, many youngsters are stabled for part, if not all, of the day, especially in bad weather. However, such management practice is not the best for psychological development of the horse as isolation can lead to behavioural problems and such horses are also prone to obesity. An alternative which goes some way to solving the problem of isolation, is to provide a field shelter (Figure 8.9) or keep youngsters barned together in groups. Youngsters can be successfully kept in this way providing time is allowed for them to develop a hierarchy, preferably in a large open field, before being confined. This system does run a higher risk of injury to weanlings so animals must be watched closely for signs of bullying. The benefits of social interaction, sunlight and *ad libitum* exercise should not be underestimated.

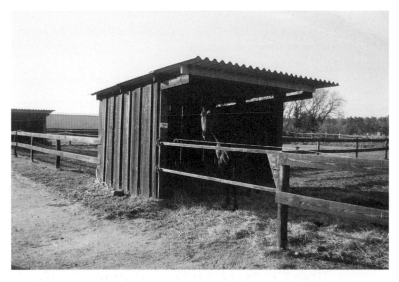

Figure 8.9 A field shelter can be provided allowing youngsters to be turned out but ensuring shelter in bad weather.

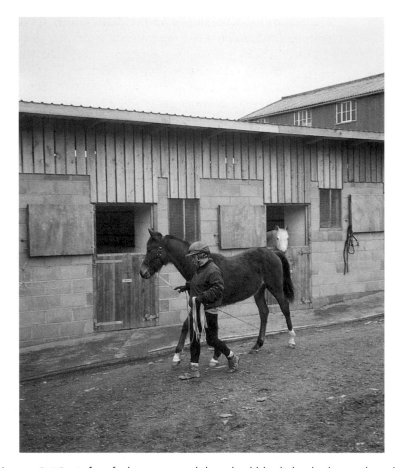

Figure 8.10 Before foals are weaned they should be halter broken and used to being handled. This eases their post-weaning management considerably. © CABI.

Weather permitting, weanlings should be turned out all the time with supplemented feed.

8.6.3 Handling

Before weaning all foals should be halter broken and be used to being handled (Figure 8.10). It is much easier to teach young foals basic manners than face a bad tempered and potentially dangerous yearling.

A well-handled youngster which is used to grooming, feet trimming, clipping, boxing etc. will be much easier to train in later life. Such an animal will have developed a confidence and respect which can be built upon in later training schedules. It is also much more likely to concentrate on the lesson in hand and, therefore, be easier to train, as he has confidence in his relationship with his handler.

When handling any youngsters it must be remembered that they can be unpredictable. By nature they are often flighty and there is no guarantee that they will always react to things in the same way. Every precaution should be taken to ensure that if the unexpected occurs no one is hurt and there is minimum panic. A youngster is very impressionable and panic or nervousness within the human handlers can easily be sensed by, and transferred to, the youngster. This can become self-perpetuating and result in an owner too frightened to handle the youngster and a nervous horse, increasingly unpredictable in its behaviour. A complete outsider is often required to break such a downward spiral.

The youngster should always be treated with constant discipline. It gains security from predictable, consistent handling, even though it will try to push the limits of behaviour. Bad habits and behaviour should be disciplined immediately with the voice. Physical punishment is not normally necessary, except in extremes, and if not carried out with care, can degenerate into a confrontational situation.

Youngsters should be taught not to bite, nip, push, barge etc. A foal should not be allowed to play with handlers. It is fun to teach a foal to 'shake hands' but when it starts to kick out in front as a yearling or older horse, this can be very dangerous. In this case, the horse cannot be blamed for doing something it was once praised for. Charging and pushing handlers, especially when leaving a stable or through a gate is potentially very dangerous. The foal should be taught to let the handler go first, and if it barges it should be halted with a short sharp tug on the lead rope.

Praise is as important as discipline and whenever a youngster does well or as it is told, it should be praised by a pat and also by voice. Throughout its handling it should get used to the human voice and certain clear commands. Initially 'whoa' is very useful to get the horse to stand still and can be used in later lungeing lessons. This is one of the most important discipline lessons to learn. As long as a horse will stand still when told, you will always have control over it. There are other commands for other actions, e.g. come to call, walk, trot on, etc. as appropriate. A horse will get used to any commands given clearly and consistently.

Initially a youngster will be very exuberant and full of energy and at this stage it may be appropriate to overlook minor bad behaviour until the basics have been achieved. It can be very demoralising for a youngster, and handler, if it is always being disciplined and can seemingly do nothing right. The less desirable behaviour can be disciplined at a later stage providing it does not get out of hand. The handler must use their common sense and assess the situation.

Beyond the basics, further handling and training will depend on the youngster's destination in life and can be geared towards a particular aim, for example, racing, breeding, showing, hacking etc. It is beyond the scope of this book to discuss the specific training of youngsters for specific disciplines.

Whatever the ultimate destiny for the youngster, exercise is always important. At about one year of age forced exercise can be introduced in the form of leading out or lungeing and provides the grounding for further training, especially in riding horses. Regular exercise also conditions horses and makes them fitter, ensuring that when training begins in earnest an initial period making them fit is not required. Training of unfit horses runs the risk of strains and sprains of unconditioned muscles and tendons, leading to a waste of time in resting injuries. A youngster which does not have enough free exercise can be very difficult to train as he will spend much of the time careering around before work can commence in earnest. Such animals are also very difficult to lunge or put in a horse walker and run a high risk of injury. A combination of free and forced exercise allows agility and physical ability to develop along with mental stimulation. Development of both mental and physical faculties is essential as a highly developed, sophisticated mental and physical state is required in many equine disciplines.

8.6.4 Nutrition

Though foals grow for the first four to five years of life until they reach maturity, the majority of growth occurs in the first year and the correct nutrition is particularly important during this period. As discussed previously nutrition must satisfy the body's requirements for growth and development, but not to excess, as this may cause obesity, which in turn puts extra strain on young limbs, tendons and the circulatory system and leads to conditions such as degenerative orthopaedic disease (DOD) (Section 7.4.4.1, p. 175), osteochondritis dissecans (OCD) and epiphysitis. In general, nutritional deficiencies in youngstock are more critical than in older animals, and so rations for weanlings should be designed very carefully.

The precise energy, protein, vitamin and mineral requirements vary with rate of growth and the youngster's expected mature weight. All horses have a nutrient requirement for maintenance; in the young animal there is an additional requirement for growth. If rapid growth is required then the nutrient intakes will be greater than for slow or moderate growth (Tables 5.2, p. 124 and 5.3, p. 126). At this stage energy is becoming the most important component of a youngster's diet (Section 8.2.4, p. 188) as the stage of development is now reaching fat deposition. Low energy levels cause slow growth rates and at the extreme can cause stunting even if the other components of the diet are appropriate. Energy levels should be increased particularly in eighteen-month-old yearlings as their requirement is higher than animals twelve to eighteen months old. For example for a youngster that will reach a mature size of 500 kg with a moderate growth rate and is not in training, daily energy requirements at six months are 15 MCal, at twelve months 18.9 MCal and at eighteen months 19.8 MCal. For horses with rapid growth and then in training the requirements are higher: 17.2 MCal at six months, 21.3 MCal at twelve months and 26.5 MCal at eighteen months (Table 5.2, p. 124). These relatively high energy levels are normally obtained by feeding concentrates, as roughage alone would not normally provide enough energy unless it was very good quality fresh pasture and moderate growth rates only are required. Roughage must, however, always be included in the diet and the diet of a twelve-month-old youngster, even one growing rapidly, must not contain more than 70% concentrate feed.

In addition to energy, protein quality and quantity continue to be essential for development (Section 8.2.4, p. 188). The daily requirement of a youngster destined to reach a mature size of 500 kg growing moderately and not in training at six months is 750 g, at twelve months is 851 and at eighteen months is 893 g. Again if more rapid growth is required and the animal is in training the daily protein requirements may reach 1200 g at eighteen months (Table 5.2, p. 124).

As might be expected, vitamin and mineral intakes even in older growing youngsters remain important. For example a six-month-old youngster with an expected 500 kg mature weight and a moderate growth rate requires 29 g/day calcium and 16 g/day phosphorus, these requirements then decline for youngsters of eighteen months of age or older to 27 g/day calcium and 15 g/day phosphorus if they are not in training (Table 5.2, p. 124). However, as with all other nutrients, if the animal is in training or rapid growth is required these nutrient requirements increase (Table 5.2, p. 124). The ratio of calcium to phosphorus is also important, a ratio of 2:1 is ideal for six-month-old youngsters, although older animals can tolerate more variation. During this growing phase other minerals such as copper, zinc and selenium, as well as Vitamins D, A and E are also important.

Within these guidelines the body condition and weight of the youngster should also be monitored and the level of feed should be altered to account for any over- or under-weight. Excessive energy levels in the feed are the main cause of obesity in youngstock and are known to contribute to conditions such as epiphysitis, structural deformities, contracted tendons, DOD (Section 7.4.4.1, p. 175) etc.

For moderately growing youngsters who are not in training, good quality fresh forage, especially over the summer months should satisfy all their requirements. However, conserved forage or restricted access to pasture will not allow all requirements to be met and so in these cases concentrates will need to be fed. As a general guide a weanling should be fed 3–4 kg/day of concentrates, split into three to four feeds. Soya bean meal is a good source of quality protein and so is popular in youngster's diets and the inclusion of a vitamin and mineral supplement, especially calcium and phosphorus, is good practice.

As always, water must not be forgotten, a continual supply of clean fresh water is essential.

8.6.5 Vaccination, parasite control, teeth and feet care

By twelve to eighteen months of age, worming and vaccination should be the same as that for the adult horse (Sections 5.5.3, p. 127 and 5.5.4, p. 129), though use of a wormer also effective against ascarids (Table 5.4, p. 128) is advised, as resistance is not fully developed until two years of age. Feet and teeth should not require specific treatment at this stage but both should be checked regularly by a qualified farrier or equine dentist to ensure that they remain in good condition and problems are identified in good time so that action can be taken.

8.7 CONCLUSION

Considerable thought should be given to the method of weaning and the handling of youngstock. Management at this young age can have long-term repercussions on the foal's physical and psychological development and so affect its ability to fulfil its potential in later life.

Index